Climax

THE POWER OF GREAT SEX

DEBRA SHADE

CLINICAL SEXOLOGIST AND MASTER SEXPERT

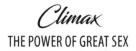

THE POWER OF GREAT SEX

ISBN: 978-1-60414-576-2

Cover art by Misha via stock.adobe.com
Cover Design by Fideli Publishing, Inc.

Published by:

Shade Publishing LLC
PO BOX 297926
Columbus, OH 43229
614-259-8370

www.ShadePublishing.com

Acknowledgements

I am forever grateful for my wife who supports me through my commitment to modern day sex education.

I am thankful for my experiences with clients that allow me to continue to improve upon my current knowledge of the orgasm. The experience is different for everyone and that makes you normal. I am an advocate for clients to take on the responsibility of their orgasm.

I am very thankful for the opportunities I am given to help people overcome the barriers to their orgasm. This book was written for the individuals who wish to learn about creating orgasms in their own way. Thank you for taking the step toward an improved orgasm.

Foreword

Erotica touches the brain in a way that pornography cannot. The way an artist like Debra Shade paints the tapestry, combines words and phrases to create mystery, and tickles and titillates the mind, it is complete magic. Using erotica to enhance the experience of orgasm is just one of the many tools that an author and sexologist like Debra Shade brings to the table in her latest work.

Debra Shade is a master of giving us just enough to then allow our imagination to step in and do the rest. Now she uses her skill as a sexologist to help augment the orgasm experience. Although orgasm is not the most important aspect of a sexual experience, it is certainly a happy ending. Now this guide can help you get there.

Dr. Rachel Ross
Founder of Dr. Rachel Institute
and host of The Doctors

Contents

Foreword...v

Preface.. xvii

Introduction.. xxi

RELATIONSHIP CONNECTION...1

Emotional 2

Social.. 3

Mental.. 3

Spiritual 4

Coupling 5

Practice 5

Put Sex on the Calendar 6

    Use any playing field...7

    Enjoy a quickie...7

    Watch Porn or an Erotic Film 8

    Employ Some Toys 8

YOUR BODY AND SEX 9

The Vagina... 10

    External..10

    Internal...10

Vagina Tests 11

    Pelvic Exam 11

    Pap Smear... 11

    Bacterial Culture... 11

    Colposcopy... 12

    Vaginal Biopsy 12

Alteration/Mutilation 12
    Labiaplasty... 12
    Clitoridectomy... 12
Vulva and Vagina Conditions................................. 12
    Vaginitis Inflammation...................................... 12
    Vaginismus... 13
    Vaginal Prolapse.. 13
Understanding Ovulation 13
    The Cervix During the Infertile Phase............... 14
    The Cervix Close to Ovulation 14
    Differences in Cervical Fluids............................. 14
    The Cervix After Ovulation 15
The Penis... 15
    Parts... 16
    Structure 16
    Size.. 17
    Normal Variations 17
    Erection.. 19
    Ejaculation.. 19
    Ejaculate Size.. 20

YOUR MIND AND SEX 21
How to Relax... 26
Understanding Orgasm 27
Orgasm Process 28
Stages of Orgasm 28
Tension & Relaxation... 29
Enjoy Stronger Orgasms 31
    A Genetal/Clitoral focused Orgasm 32
    A Deep / Full-Body orgasm,................................ 32

Release and Relax into the Orgasmic Wave 34

How to Achieve Deep Orgasm 35

How Do You Tell the Difference Between
    These Orgasms? 35

A Technique for Pre-Orgasmic Vulva Owners 36

EROGENOUS ZONES 38

Yoni Massage 39

Clitoral Orgasm 39

Vaginal Orgasm 41

A-spot 42

Deep Spot Orgasm 44

U-spot Orgasm 44

Breast Orgasm 45

Oral Orgasm 47

Skin Orgasm 48

Mental Orgasm 49

G-spot Orgasm 49

Megagasm 51

BIGGER BODIED SEX 53

Modification is Key 54

Cause for Concern 54

Positions with Modification 55

Doggy Style 55
Cowgirl 55
Spooning 55
Leg Glider 56
Thigh Tide 56

Butterfly 56
Deep Impact 57

What If the Giver Is Bigger?...................................**57**
Building Self Confidence...**59**

ALL YOU NEED TO KNOW ABOUT STRAP-ONS 59

History **60**
Harness Materials...**61**
   Synthetic 61
   O-ring harness 61
   Leather 61
   Cloth...61
   Plastic 61
   Clear Plastic Harness...62
   Latex, Rubber, PVC 62
   Molded Straps 62

Harness Types..**63**
   A two-strap harness...63
   Three-strap 63
   Corsets and other clothing items...........................63
   Body locations...64
   Vacuum Seal 64
   Strapless 65
   O-Ring Harness with Wide-Base Dildo 65

Specialty Functions **66**
   Inflatable Enema Nozzle..66
   Dildos..66
   Standard...66
   Probe 66
   G-Spot and Prostate 67
   Penis Extensions 67

Upon Objects 67
Vibrating and Rotating 68
Double penetration 68

EXTERNAL STIMULATION **70**
Jelly-coated vibrating egg..................................... 70
Vibrators 70

INTERNAL STIMULATION **71**
Double-ended attachments 71
Strap-on harness with dual internal plugs............... 71
Double-ended/sided hands and strap free dildos....... 71

WHAT TO DO WITH THE REST OF HIM **73**
Imagination 74
Abdomen and Navel 74
Spine 74
Fingers 74
Armpits 75
Arms 75
Hair 75
The Feet in General.. 76
Toes 76
Butt Cheek 76
The Philtrum 77
Inner Thigh 77
Bottom Lips 78
The Outside of their Lower Lip 78
V-Lines.. 78
Neck 79

Nipples 79

The Dip Under Their Ankle 80

Lower Back 81

Earlobes 81

The Raphe 80

Perineum 81

Shaft 81

The Head of the Penis 81

The Seam of the Testicles 82

Frenulum 82

ANAL ORGASM **83**

What You Should Know 84

Anal Play and the Law 85

The Anus 86

Play Safely 86

For Teens 87

Lubes 88

Anal Toys 88

Anal Beads 89

Butt Plugs 89

Anal Toy Materials 90

What to Avoid 90

Clean Your Butt and Your Toys 91

Enemas and Douches 91

Sharing Your Anal Toys 92

Toy Features 93

YOUR HEALTH AND SEX **94**

PC Muscle 96

The Problem Could Be Medical.......................................97

Benefits of Eros Therapy Clitoral Device include:............98

Female Sexual Dysfunction (FSD) 98

Various Definitions of Female Sexual Dysfunction 98

Sexual Desire Disorders **98**

Hypoactive sexual desire disorder 98

Sexual aversion disorder...99

Sexual Arousal Disorder..99

Orgasmic Disorder..99

Sexual Pain Disorders 99

SEX POSITIONS **101**

Missionary **102**

Doggy Style **103**

The CAT **103**

Mountain Climber.. **103**

Quickie Fix.. **103**

Standing Tiger, Crouching Dragon **104**

Wheelbarrow Standing **104**

The Ballet Dancer **104**

Stand and Deliver **104**

Butter Churner.. **104**

The Flatiron **105**

The G-Whiz... **105**

The Pretzel **105**

One Up.. **106**

Heir to the Throne... **106**

David Copperfield 106

The Cowgirl.. 106

Reverse Cowgirl 107

Pole Position... 107

The Hot Seat 107

Face Off... 108

The Lazy Man.. 108

Spoon, facing 108

Spork.. 108

Spoon 109

The Spider 109

Snow Angel 109

The X Position 110

The Elevator 110

Cowgirl 69.. 110

Hovering Butterfly 110

Swiss Ball Blitz 111

Rest Room Attendant.. 111

SEXUAL HEALTH SAFETY 112

Myths 112

**SEXUALLY TRANSMITTED INFECTIONS
AND DISEASES**.. 117

Trichomoniasis (Trich) 117

Scabies.. 118

Syphilis.. 119

Hepatitis A-E 120

Molluscum Contagiosum 121

Pubic Lice... 121

HPV (Human Papilloma Virus............................ 122

HIV and AIDS 123

Gonorrhea (The Clap) 123

Herpes... 124

Vaginal Yeast 125

Vaginosis (Bv) 126

Yeast In Men (Balanitis) 127

Pelvic Inflammatory Disease (Pid) 128

Chlamydia.. 129

HPV(Warts) 131

KEEPING IT SEXY **132**

Things to Do 132

16 Days and Dozens of Ways
  to Reignite Romantic Love 135

REFERENCES **143**

ABOUT THE AUTHOR **145**

Preface

As an orgasm coach, I spend a lot of time helping my clients reach their best orgasmic experience. I guide them through barriers to the orgasm. Using cognitive behavior theory exercises and talk therapy, I have been successful in getting individuals to the point of finding their best experience.

I wasn't always a Clinical Sexologists and Master Sexpert. The process of becoming who I am today came from my love of writing. I wrote a book that I thought was erotica. After several signings, I realized that my audience included folks who were embarrassed to hear the content and those who were so intrigued they stayed after to ask questions about the sex I had read to them. Turns out it was more literary porn than erotica. However, the questions revealed that people needed to know that there is a world of sexual pleasure that they can tap into. Orgasms are beneficial to your health. You should have them frequently. Because of this, you should gain modern day sex education that appreciates the orgasm.

Sex education that does not include the orgasm has left a society of individuals who have never experienced an orgasm or have never been able to repeat their best orgasm. These conversations got me more and more interested in sharing the knowledge that I had about sex education. I started the educational path to become certified. This certification allows me to offer services to clients that they have never been exposed to. I enjoy what I do. I started offering workshops and seminars nationwide and fell in love with my success rate. I work with clients all over the world, regardless of orientation or gender. This allows me to help as many people as I can. I am invited to speak at conferences, festivals, expos, and seminars. This allows me to reach a wider audience.

I am hopeful that I can reach even more through this book. This book is intended to educate individuals on topics of pleasure. Within the first chapter, you will find information on the benefits of your connection with your mate in a relationship. Understanding the importance of a connection and orgasm. Body, mind, and health all play major roles in sex. It's important to understand your body and be pleased with it. Your body image can alter your ability to achieve a full-body orgasm. I provide positions for pleasure for all, with a special piece for bigger bodied individuals.

A great experience can't be had if you have sexual health issues on the table. I discuss painful intercourse, the need to control your PC muscle and medical issues that may prevent orgasm. This information can help you understand the orgasm. I take a detailed look at the process of orgasm and types of orgasms that vulva owners can have and of course, orgasms for penis owners. You can't have an orgasm conversation without the use of sex toys such as strap-ons. Knowing how to put a great harness to use is priceless. It raises the bar with sexual pleasure, allowing for many variations of use.

Which brings me to the benefits of stimulating erogenous zones. The body holds so many areas that can be stimulated to the point of arousal and/or orgasm. These are great tips to know to build and maintain foreplay techniques. Foreplay is needed to prepare the body for orgasm.

Finally, I wrap up with a chapter on keeping it sexy within a relationship that will give you a plan to maintain the sexual connection in long term relationships. It is my hope that you will be able to take the knowledge within this book to develop your best sexual experiences. Claim your orgasm and determine for yourself what that looks like. Your orgasm is your responsibility. Get to a point where you can tell your mate what that looks like and then be open to receiving the best orgasm of your life.

Introduction

You have just picked up a key to your best orgasm. As an Orgasm Coach, I spend most of my time coaching individuals and couples through barriers to their orgasms. It is not always easy to have an orgasm. Whether you are a penis owner or a vulva owner, your orgasm experience is your own and could include complications. We all have different relationships with orgasms.

I have had the pleasure of mastering achieving an orgasm, specifically a squirting orgasm, one of the most sought-after orgasms. I have the pleasure of helping people understand their orgasm. How to achieve, enjoy and provide orgasm are all lessons life rarely teaches you without trial and error. This book will discuss the process of orgasm and leave you with skills and techniques to become an orgasm master.

Permit yourself to read this book. Open yourself to its content and your ability to achieve a great orgasmic experience every time. Read it with your partner and learn how to give and receive orgasm together. Commitment is key when I talk with my clients. I need them to be open to the work it takes to clear the 'brain plate' and be free to enjoy sex.

Commit to practicing the techniques described within this book as it may take you out of your comfort zone and it may also require you to work on your stamina, attention span, or your relationship with pleasure. Let it challenge you, grow and find yourself having your best orgasm from solo play or with a mate.

Relationship Connection

One of the most sought-after experiences among humans is connection. We want to feel wanted, supported, loved, appreciated, and desired. With connection, you free yourself from loneliness and replace it with joy. Connections happen when partners have time to be together in fun, loving ways.

Communication is key in every sexual situation you will find yourself in. Consent literally is an ongoing conversation that you can retract at any time. Telling your partner what you want and what will give you the most pleasure takes open communication. It is encouraging to have a conversation at the start and throughout the experience. Sometimes it can be done by body language, but to avoid miscommunication, speak up for yourself.

The more quality and quantify connection you have, the better chance you have of being successful in your relationship.

Even in some instances, one-night stands can include communication that will set up the evening for the most success, and it's even more important to have that form of communication in long term relationships. The communication is the glue that keeps the relationship together.

Connection in long term relationship is everything. Infatuation, lust, love, and communication are all parts of the formula needed to build a strong foundation that can withstand challenges. In the beginning phases of the relationship, you question how connected you are. What connects you? Is it beyond physical attraction?

You need to have something beyond physical attraction to stay connected fully within your relationship. Look at the depth and width of the connection that you have. Are you also connected mentally, socially, emotionally and/or spiritually? Ask yourself how many of these areas you share a bond.

EMOTIONAL

Being open to share your feelings with each other, shows a healthy emotional connection. This means that you have to be vulnerable with each other. Be emotionally expressive. Share your fear, loneliness, shame, and/or sadness with them. When the feel-good chemicals in your brain start to fade, you may find yourself with less ecstatic feelings for your mate. This is when the connection that you have created can be maintained.

For this to work, the connection must be reciprocal. You may not be able to create a healthy relationship if you are not on the same page. Determine the expected life of the relationship and build your connection with that foundation. Having open, authentic conversations will help you figure out if there is a true emotional connection.

To maintain this connection, always reflect and lean on the foundation created by your vulnerability with each other. Keep communication at the top of your relationship tools list. Checking in with each other, supporting each other, be romantic and always be true to yourself. This gives you permission to communicate and ask for what you seek in a relationship.

SOCIAL

Today we are inundated in social media sites. It's a great way to keep up with your friends, make plans even. A great way to meet new people and to network via the many groups within the sites. The way that you interact socially can affect the connection you have in a relationship. It helps to have similar traits in the way you use social media.

Sharing mutual interest, activities, hobbies, and lifestyle can help you build a healthy social connection. Do you spend time enjoying each other's company? Are you active with their friends and family? Create these types of connections to have a healthy relationship.

How you relate to each other determines your social connection. Look at how you interact with each other and the outside world. If your friends as well as lovers, you have a combination of balance that will support your connection with your mate.

MENTAL

Your open communication will help you in this area. Mentally supporting someone means you have to be mentally strong. Be sure you create and implement a system of wellness so that you are mentally present in your relationship. Mediate, take walks, do yoga, write, or call a friend are all great ways of mental care you can use.

The thing to remember is that connection you have that allows you to be vulnerable with each other. You must be able to support each other when one is triggered. Hurt, fear and sadness exist for those with trauma. Instead of reacting to your partner's triggers with your own anger or withdrawal, learn to be there with compassion and care for one another.

It does not mean that you need to own your partner's feelings. Just honor them. Show a level of support that will help them deal with their painful feelings. A true connection can be made when you use compassion for each other's wounds and vulnerabilities. This of course, will allow you to maintain well-being as well. Getting the reciprocal support from your mate. Sometimes it is necessary to seek therapy, coaching or facilitation to overcome what stops a person from moving forward and building strong connections.

Remain present; nothing disconnects partners more than speaking to someone who is not listening or paying you any attention. This is a sign of disconnect and an area that can be improved. Be present when you are with your partner, look at them, nod or show facial expressions that let them know that you are listening and honoring what they are saying.

If you happen to find yourself preoccupied when you are with your partner, then do some mental work around why you are avoiding making a mental connection with your partner. If you want to maintain the connection, you need to learn to be present for your partner.

SPIRITUAL

Have you ever heard the saying "the family that prays together stays together"? There is some truth to this. Whether you are praying to the same entity, you can support each other spiritually. You can allow them to be connected to their spiritual endeavors and you to yours. Not having the same faith is not an excuse to not connect on a spiritual level with your partner. Connect first with yourself; you cannot be disconnected from yourself and support someone else. When you are comfortable in your beliefs, you can be strong and capable in the relationship. You will connect with your partner because you wanted to share your love.

COUPLING

You may need to be able to create balance to maintain a healthy relationship. You may be smarter, have more money, but you think so similarly; you have shared values and find that you want the relationship. You want to build a connection and want to be in a fulfilling relationship, and you think this person can provide that for you.

While physical chemistry is really important, you have to be sure it's not temporary. Monitor the relationship as you move forward for signs of connection and stability. If your relationship is lacking in other areas, you may worry about connecting on other levels. Coupling means you are willing to do the work on all levels to create a solid connection.

When you feel like you are meant to be together, you have met your kindred spirit. If you feel a deeper connection, you may be with each other for a reason. Connection is multi-layered, depending on who you are and what you need in a relationship.

PRACTICE

Here is what you do. You first must be open to learning. Consistently we are either intent to learn about love and truth or the intent to protect against pain with some form of controlling behavior. This closes your heart and disconnects you from yourself, your partner, and others. When the heart is open, you can connect. You just cannot connect to a closed heart. Choose the intent to learn when you're with your partner.

Take the time to focus on what you value in your partner; sure, there are things that you don't like, but don't fester on those. Allow your love and support to be reflected back to you. Your needs may make the bad not so bad. It all depends on how you value the relationship. When you do inner work and learn to love and value yourself, then you can also value the essence of your partner. Be careful falling back on controlling behaviors. Learn protective behaviors. Behaviors that will allow you to live with an open heart because you are protected from triggers.

You are your essence, soul self, or true self; this is likely what you fell in love with when you first fell for your partner. Focus on your partner's wounded behaviors that come from their fear and you will create distance. Allow them to process; you be there to hold their hand and that is building connection. Focus on their great qualities.

Do something fun; making time to be together in a fun and relaxed way are opportunities for connection. Watching a funny show, hold hands and talk, cook together, create something, or share something interesting together. Take every opportunity to keep things fresh and fun. Remember the days when you sat and talked forever? You can recreate that, and you can enjoy a life together when you employ awesome ways to connect.

Very high on the list of things to try to build connection is supporting what brings your partner joy. You know how much easier it is to keep your heart open when you are feeling joyful. Supporting each other in what you each enjoy will make the times when they are out with friends or doing something alone non-threating. Connection is everything in healthy relationships.

PUT SEX ON THE CALENDAR

Often, we don't have sex because life is busy, we can't find a mate, and it's offered at the wrong time of the month. Whatever the reason, sex may fall by the wayside if you do not schedule it. This is not to say that spontaneity goes out the window, it just ensures that you will be having sex at some point in the very near future.

Don't pick a holiday, a birthday, or the same location each time. Determine what location and time works for both of you. You want to be sure that you take away the distraction of your to-do list because it's on your list. You're free to enjoy the experience.

Start foreplay early

You don't have to wait until it's time to get busy before you began to turn each other on. Start as early in the day as possible. Wake each other up with a sexy whisper, call, or text just to let them know you are thinking of them. Don't be vulgar (unless that is wanted foreplay) but use sexy words and phrases. Brush against them at the sink or hold hands as you part ways. Whatever feels sexy to you may very well feel sexy for your mate. Engage them early and keep them aroused all day long.

Use any playing field

Utilize all the square footage of your home for sex. Not just the bedroom. Use the coffee table before a dinner party and keep her smiling throughout the event. You have heard what siting on the washer or dryer will add to the experience. Bathrooms and stairs allow you to bend, stand or kneel in various positions. Of course, you can use the sofa, lean them over the sofa facedown. Place a scarf under her so that it rubs the genitals as you thrust. Take it outside. The air, smells and sounds add excitement to having sex outdoors.

Enjoy a quickie

Individuals don't always need 10 or 20 minutes of foreplay. A quickie is just that. You must be able to get your mate turned on and engaged within a very short period of time. Kiss seductively unexpectantly against a cabinet and raise their skirt or cup their ass. Take the time to dry hump on the sofa until your reaching for each other with heart-pounding adrenaline. There is no better way to start the day than the spontaneous erotic rush of a quickie.

Watch Porn or an Erotic Film

Watching other people have sex can trigger lusty thoughts about your partner and spice up your sex life. Have a heart to heart talk about how they really feel about erotic movies and porn in general. Pick films in which the actors look more physically like you or your partner so that the body types are ones that turn you on. Be careful of reenacting what you see, be inspired but be careful of your safety as you have sex.

Employ Some Toys

Cock Rings, vibrators, dildos, or pumps can enhance the entire experience. Most vulva owners concentrate on their clit, penetrating only when ready to climax. Stroke the outer labia and clit during foreplay. Gyrating along with these pleasure points by increasing pressure will push the desire to the tipping point so that when you penetrate, you will deliver an orgasm-inducing thrust.

G-Spot stimulators are toys that target the spongy, sensitive area in the upper vaginal wall. A G-Spot orgasm comes from strategic pressure not size. Thus, add pressure with each thrust and enter when they are on their back with their knees resting on their chest.

The Rabbit Vibrator rubs both sides of the clitoris. Thus, use your index and ring fingers to rub the sides. Simultaneously stroke the top of the clit with a middle finger, completing the trick to send them over the edge.

The Classic Vibrator has multiple speeds that massage nerve-rich erogenous spots as it intensifies. Thus, a little change is good. Start slow, gentile and use broad strokes with your finger and tongue. Build toward a climax, instead of rapidly changing techniques and intensity.

Your Body and Sex

If you don't know your body, you are not going to be able to enjoy a fulfilling sex life. There are many reasons why you should work on knowing your body and all its pleasure points. The biggest reason for having a great relationship in your body is so that you can openly share it with others. Body mindfulness is a great way to learn to love your body. Learn to love every curve and dimple you own. When you learn to do that, you free yourself and give permission to allow your body pleasure.

Your body is equipped with genitals that allow you to experience orgasms, for some, orgasms are the name of the game. The star of the show. For others, orgasm is not an interest. I want to address those individuals that seek orgasm. It does take some inner work to get yourself to the point where you are happy with your body enough to share it with your partner. If you put in that work, you can get to the point of having a great orgasm.

The connection is both mental and physical. Taking thought distortions off the table allows you to enjoy every moment of sex. It allows you to be present, to participate and to work in unison with their partners to have their best experience. This distortion may include a lack of understanding of the female anatomy. When I use the term female,

I am addressing vulva owners. Tied to current labeling of male or female, I am limited in description that is all inclusive. Bottom line, this information is for you if you seek to have great orgasms.

Coming up, I am going to break down the genitals for you. I want you to get friendly with them, feel and caress them and get to know them. You can ask for what you need by knowing what it takes for yourself. Let's look at the anatomy of the vagina, take note of the parts that are orgasmic. Take note of those areas for your own body. Take time to get to know yourself; your relationship with your body makes a difference.

THE VAGINA

I encourage you to take a moment and look at and examine your vagina. Get familiar with it in hopes that you will fall in love with it. You will become committed to taking care of it. The vagina is made up of both external and internal parts.

External

The first thing you will see is the clitoris. It is located at the top of the vulva and varies in size and sensitivity, most have over eight thousand nerve endings.

Right below the clitoris is the urethra opening. This is the tiny hole your pee comes out of.

The next part is the vaginal opening; this is right below the urethra opening. This is where your menstrual flow and babies come out of.

The opening of the rectum is the anus. The anus is connected to the vulva by an area called the perineum.

Internal

The vagina is a tube connected to the vulva via the cervix and uterus. It can receive things within it and push things out.

Cervix is between the vagina and uterus. It is a doughnut looking tube that can be felt behind the vagina.

Fallopian tubes are two narrow tubes that carry eggs from the ovaries to the uterus; it is also where sperm swim up.

The uterus is where babies grow. It is a muscular organ that is the size of a small fist.

Skene's Gland are also known as female prostate glands. They are on each side of the urethral opening and release a fluid during ejaculation.

Fimbriae are tiny tubes at the end of the fallopian tubes that push sperm toward eggs.

The ovaries are where the female eggs are stored. They release several different hormones that make drastic changes at menopause.

Hymen is the thin tissue that goes across part of the vagina opening. It is usually torn the first time something penetrates it.

VAGINA TESTS

Pelvic Exam — An exam of the entire reproductive organs. This is a yearly exam that can be done in a regular checkup. Symptoms of a vaginal condition may require an exam as well. The exam only lasts for minutes where your doctor checks your vulva, vagina, cervix, ovaries, uterus, rectum, and pelvis for any abnormalities.

Pap Smear — You and your doctor will determine when to begin Pap testing, which shall be performed when an abnormality exists. Most doctors recommend starting testing when you start your period.

Bacterial Culture — The specialist will look at multiple microbial organisms under laboratory conditions. They use the results of the culture to make diagnosis and suggest care.

Colposcopy — This is a fairly safe procedure. Its purpose is to remove tissue to be examined by the laboratory.

Vaginal Biopsy — Sometimes, a vaginal biopsy is needed. This is done through a colposcopy. If an unusual area of cells is found, a tissue sample will be taken and tested.

ALTERATION/MUTILATION

Labiaplasty — A plastic surgery procedure for altering the labia minora and the labia majora, the folds of skin surrounding the human vulva.

Women have taken control over their own bodies and have decided to get labiaplasty. Sometimes, a person may have feelings of disconnect between their vulva appearance and the way it is mentally received. Alternation gives them the power to move forward and claim their sexual health.

Clitoridectomy — In some cultures, the clitoris is amputated to deny sexual pleasure. It is also known as a clitorectomy. It is rarely used as a therapeutic procedure. It is often performed on intersex newborns.

VULVA AND VAGINA CONDITIONS

We must pay close attention to our vulva and vagina hygiene and care. Doing so will help prevent infections and pain. Look for unusual changes in the vaginal discharge as a sign that something may be wrong.

A lump or sore on the vulva that itches may be a rare form of cancer which is treated with surgery as needed. Not everyone will need to have surgery. Every lump or sore should be taken seriously and discussed with your primary doctor. Below is a list of conditions you should monitor for the vulva and the vagina.

Vaginitis Inflammation — Vaginitis is an inflammation of the vagina. It may lead to discharge, pain, and itching. It usually develops when the normal balance of vaginal bacteria is altered. Reduced estrogen levels after menopause and some skin disorders can also cause vaginitis.

Vaginismus — Vaginismus is when the muscles around the opening of the vagina involuntarily contract. This makes sex or sex related activity that involves penetration very painful or impossible.

Vaginal Prolapse — When the upper portion of the vagina loses its shape and sags or drops down into the vaginal canal or outside of the vagina. It is repairable with surgery and can be in conjunction with prolapse of the urethra, rectum, bladder, or small bowel.

UNDERSTANDING OVULATION

The cervix is the passageway into your uterus, and you can feel it change throughout your cycle. Checking on these changes can help you determine where in your cycle you are. Just as each body is unique, so too are their signs of ovulation.

During different phases of your cycle, your cervix will behave differently. There are two main phases for the cervix — the infertile phase and the period where the cervix is approaching ovulation. Most women have a menstrual cycle of 28 days, but it is also reasonable to have anything from 21 to 35 days. Some have irregular menstrual cycles, which can significantly affect their chances of conceiving.

There are those who have more than one menstrual period a month (shorter menstrual cycles) and those who have longer menstrual cycles with fewer menstrual periods a year. The cervix position and firmness changes throughout the menstrual cycle. You can check the position and texture of your cervix by inserting your clean middle finger into your vagina up to at least your middle knuckle. Notice how it feels, and then continue checking your cervix throughout your cycle.

The Cervix During the Infertile Phase

During this period, the cervix seems to be elongated and off-center so that it can rest against the vaginal wall. The cervix will feel firm, similar to the tip of your nose. Furthermore, the opening will feel dry. Finally, the cervix is easily reached at this time, as it lies low in the vagina.

The Cervix Close to Ovulation

Increasing estrogen levels force the cervix further up into the vagina the closer you get to ovulation. As a result, the cervix comes across as positioned more centrally in the vagina. It also appears shorter and straighter in addition to feeling softer. Rather than feeling like the tip of a nose, the cervix now feels like your lower lip.

Differences in Cervical Fluids

The role of your cervix is to create fertile cervical fluid during ovulation to help the sperm travel easily, as well as to block the entrance to the uterus when you are not fertile. After menstruation, you will experience little or no discharge. Your first cervical discharge will appear moist or sticky, will be either white or cream colored, and continue for a few more days. As you get closer to ovulation, you will notice the consistency of your cervical mucus changes. It becomes thinner and less sticky. The amount of cervical mucus will also increase. This thin cervical mucus will gradually increase until you hit your 'cervical mucus peak.' When you are at your most fertile, your cervical mucus looks like 'egg whites' and is indicative that you are about to ovulate. This discharge will be slippery and colorless and indicates your best chance at conception.

The Cervix After Ovulation

Once ovulation is complete, the cervix will generally return to its infertile state within 24 to 48 hours. Since each person's body is different, you have to remember that the average cycle does not apply to everyone and if changes in the cervix are going to be used to aid in conception, it is essential to figure out when you ovulate accurately.

THE PENIS

Ever wonder what mysteries the penis holds? Understanding the structure of the penis can lead to giving and receiving better orgasms. Let's cover the parts of the penis, its structure, size, normal variations including erection, erection angle and ejaculation. You will be able to use this information to perform better blow jobs, hands jobs and various positions.

Different than most other mammals, it has no erectile bone. Instead, it is engorged with blood to reach its erect state. In its flaccid (relaxed/soft/limp) state, the shaft of the penis feels like a dense sponge encased in very smooth eyelid-type skin. The tip or glans of the penis is darker in color and covered by the foreskin if present.

In its fully erect state, the shaft of the penis is rigid, with the skin tightly stretched. The glans of the erect penis has the feel of a raw mushroom. The erect penis may be straight or curved and may point at an upward or downward angle, or straight ahead. It may also tend to lean to the left or right.

Parts

Some may believe that the penis is the shaft and balls. The penis has been studied and parts have been identified as they have a different purpose. Within the parts there are areas that we know cause pleasure which increases the blood flow to the area, and we know that this brings on the erection.

Root of the penis. It is the attached part, consisting of the bulb of penis in the middle and the crus of penis, one on either side of the bulb. It lies within the superficial perineal pouch.

Body of the penis. It has two surfaces: posterosuperior in the erect penis and ventral or urethral (facing downwards and backwards in the flaccid penis). The ventral surface is marked by a groove in a lateral direction.

Epithelium of the penis consists of the shaft skin, the foreskin, and the preputial mucosa on the inside of the foreskin and covering the glans penis. The epithelium is not attached to the underlying shaft, so it is free to glide back and forth.

Structure

The human penis is made up of three columns of tissue, two corpora cavernosa lie next to each other on the top and one corpus spongiosum lies between them on the bottom.

The enlarged and bulbous-shaped end of the shaft forms the glans penis, which supports the foreskin, a loose fold of skin that in adults can retract to expose the glans. The area on the underside of the penis, where the foreskin is attached, is called the frenum. The rounded base of the glans is called the corona. The perineal raphe is the noticeable line along the underside of the penis.

The urethra, which is the last part of the urinary tract, crosses the corpus spongiosum, and its opening, known as the meatus, this lies on the tip of the glans penis. It is a passage for both urine and for the ejaculation of semen. Sperm are produced in the testes and stored in the attached epididymis. During ejaculation, sperm are propelled up two ducts that pass over and behind the bladder. Fluids are added by the seminal vesicles and the vas deferens turns into the ejaculatory ducts, which join the urethra inside the prostate gland. The prostate as well as the glands, add further secretions, and the semen is expelled through the penis.

The raphe is the visible ridge between the lateral halves of the penis running from the opening of the urethra across the scrotum to the area between scrotum and anus.

Size

While results vary across studies, the consensus is that the average erect human penis is approximately 5.1–5.9 in length, with 95% of adult males falling within the interval 4.2–7.5 in. Neither age nor size of the flaccid penis accurately predicted erectile length. Stretched length is most closely correlated with erect length. The average penis size is slightly larger than the median size.

Length of the flaccid penis does not necessarily correspond to the length of the erect penis; some smaller flaccid penises grow much longer, while some larger flaccid penises grow comparatively less.

The longest officially documented human penis was found by physician Robert Latou Dickinson. It was 13.5 in long and 6.26 in around.

Normal Variations

The most common form of genital alteration is circumcision, removal of part or all of the foreskin for various cultural, religious and, more rarely, medical reasons. There is controversy surrounding circumcision to date. The debate includes the fact that parents get to make such an important decision for the penis born individual. The alteration is considered "normal" for most. The area is kept clean by pulling the skin back and cleaning the head and frenum of the penis.

Individuals are born with abnormalities such as pearly penile papules. This is a common anatomical variation. It is believed to be the vestigial remnants of penis spines. Many may experience skin tightens that does not allow the foreskin to be pulled back. These are based on genetics and are identified at birth. Some can be corrected as it may negatively affect your sex life and some you will need to accept as a normal variation of the penis.

Pearly penile papules are raised bumps of somewhat paler color around the base of the glans which typically develop in men aged 20 to 40. They may be mistaken for warts but are not harmful or infectious and do not require treatment.

Fordyce spots are small, raised, yellowish-white spots 1–2 mm in diameter that may appear on the penis, which again are common and not infectious.

Sebaceous prominences are raised bumps similar to Fordyce's spots on the shaft of the penis, located at the sebaceous glands and are normal.

Phimosis is an inability to retract the foreskin fully. It is normal and harmless in infancy and pre-pubescence, occurring in about 8% of boys at age 10.

Curvature: few penises are completely straight, with curves commonly seen in all directions. Sometimes the curve is very prominent, but it rarely inhibits sexual intercourse. Curvature as great as 30° is considered normal and medical treatment is rarely considered unless the angle exceeds 45°. Changes to the curvature of a penis may be caused by Peyronie's disease.

Erection

An erection is the stiffening and rising of the penis, which occurs during sexual arousal, though it can also happen in non-sexual situations. Spontaneous erections frequently occur during adolescence due to friction with clothing, nervousness, a full bladder or large intestine, hormone fluctuations, and undressing in a nonsexual situation.

It is also normal for erections to occur during sleep and upon waking. The primary physiological mechanism that brings about erection is the autonomic dilation of arteries supplying blood to the penis, which allows more blood to fill the three spongy erectile tissue chambers in the penis, causing it to lengthen and stiffen. The now-engorged erectile tissue presses against and constricts the veins that carry blood away from the penis. More blood enters than leaves the penis until an equilibrium is reached where an equal volume of blood flows into the dilated arteries and out of the constricted veins; a constant erectile size is achieved at this equilibrium. The scrotum will usually tighten during erection. Erection facilitates sexual intercourse though it is not essential for various other sexual activities.

Ejaculation

Ejaculation is the ejecting of semen from the penis and is usually accompanied by orgasm, although it does not always. A series of muscular contractions delivers semen containing sperm from the penis. It is usually the result of sexual stimulation, which may include prostate stimulation. Rarely, it is due to prostatic disease. Ejaculation may occur spontaneously during sleep, known as a wet dream.

Anejaculation is the condition of being unable to ejaculate.

Ejaculation has two phases: *emission* and *ejaculation proper*. The emission phase of the ejaculatory reflex is under control of the sympathetic nervous system, while the ejaculatory phase is under control of a spinal reflex at the level of the spinal nerves S2–4 via the pudendal nerve. Sexual stimulation precedes ejaculation and a refractory period is needed after.

Ejaculate Size

The number of sperm in any given ejaculate varies from one ejaculate to another. This variation is hypothesized to be an attempt to eliminate, if not reduce, their sperm competition. A male will alter the number of sperm they inseminate according to their perceived level of sperm competition, inseminating a higher number of sperm if they suspect a greater level of competition from other mates.

This information can help you use your tongue, fingers, or feet to stimulate the penis to orgasm. Understanding penis angle will aid you in finding comfortable positions that are best for you and your mate. The more comfortable you both are, the more likely you will be able to reach orgasm without obstruction.

Your Mind and Sex

Head space means the time you spend during or before intercourse worrying about the grocery list, the babysitter, bills, your body, your sexual skillset and/or the list goes on. A great way to get out of your head space is to breathe easy as foreplay begins and relax through and into the actual intercourse. Stay present with your lover. If you find yourself straying to a to-do list, stop, feel your mate, feel the sheets or couch, feel the hairs raising all over your body. Reconnect to the sex that is happening right now. Believe in the FACT that your mate would not be with you if they did not like your body type, intellect, sexual acceptance, looks. Have faith in yourself that for this experience, this one right now, it's the best it can be to give and receive pleasure.

I bet you won't be surprised to read that I am a huge advocate for clearing your mind before sex. Mindfulness is huge when it comes to enjoying a satisfying sex life. You must find a way to be within your mind without allowing your mind to play tricks on you. Nasty tricks that will stifle your sex life.

You may have been told that you have the "power" to control many things with your confidence. From mates to promotions, we can simple "be" and all our individual wants will be answered.

I am sure that I am not alone in saying that this "IS NOT" the case. We must "work" hard at what we want.

From jobs, neighborhoods, partners, sex; everything takes work, takes commitment and most importantly, "fuel". Our own personal source of power, what pushes us forward, what gets us wet. We need to learn how to embrace and use our own personal "fuel". It is "my" belief that we can't do that until we embrace our inner selves and be "OK" with what we see when we look in the mirror.

Even if that mirror is your coworkers or the cutie from the bar. How they perceive us determines how we feel, how we wear our hair, how often we trade, barter and bargain on the sexiest shoes, the cutest dress. They determine how we react to them!

They reflect what they see or what we want them to see in their responses and reaction to us.

When was the last time you told somebody off about one of your fashion choices? From your head to your toes, you garner a reaction and require reaction. The issue is within us. But so is the answer. To acquire this fuel, we need to first embrace ourselves, find out our weakness and strengths when it comes to self-perception, and how you want to be perceived by others.

For most, this could mean stepping outside of some major comfort zones. Such as dressing more seductive or less seductive or more business, purposeful. After getting dressed for the day, do you feel energized from what you see to go to work with a smile, wash cloths, dust, clean, cook etc.?

This isn't good/bad. What I want to relay is that all we need to simply be, is an ability to harness our own fuel. Liking what you see in the mirror and starting your day this way is most impactful and directly tied to your level of productivity and mind power.

Some may call it confidence. Confidence is an overall mood that we get in, when looking into your mirror and seeing exactly what you want others to see/perceive. Depending on the level of satisfaction you separately experience, we can channel the energy and turn it into fuel. Fuel to affirm our inner or outer beauty. Fuel to look and accept our bodies, our hair, smile, and even teeth.

This self-reflection and alternations ought to result in changes. Use your fuel to become the exact person you want to be. Use it to determine exactly what it is you want, what you want to do, where you want to go, where you want to be, etc. Make changes as you see fit.

Have you gotten that feeling of denial when you found out that those hotties were not talking about you, but rather your friend, who happened to be more confident? Everyone has been through it before. Those days are long over if you're ready to revamp your style and turn everyone's heads. No matter your hair color, skin color, body shape, or eye color, you too can become in touch with your confidence today. But remember- don't ever try to change yourself and who you are for someone else. It's not worth it!

Confidence isn't defined and depicted in one shell. It is self-confidence. Period. It is a matter of how you burn your source of fuel. It may mean learning how to gaze intensely. Maintain eye contact without appearing creepy. Do the lopsided grin. Travel your gaze up and down the body of the person of interest (again without appearing creepy). Let them feel that you are checking them out and that you like what you are seeing.

It may mean learning how to flirt. Hold their gaze, stare at their lips, wink, be cool, stay calm, be relaxed and comfortable. Flirting is fun and harmless and a fantastic way to be seductive. Keep that mysterious air about you. People are attracted to something puzzling.

Let go of resistance and a fear of change whether it be a change in your personality, dress, or favorite place to hang out. Once you decided that you want to embrace your sensual side and get comfortable in it. It can indeed be a sensual friend.

Let's talk about things that you can do to meet your confident side, one small change at a time!

Show your style. Whether it resembles someone else — Beyoncé, Roseanne, Jonathan — show your style. What a boring place earth would be if we were all the same. Exhibit the parts of you that are special to you and you alone.

Look in the mirror. Pick your features of which you are most satisfied with, and show them off with clothes, makeup, or accessories. If you seem to know what you've got, others will get the message and notice you for what you have.

Gain confidence. Confidence involves a belief in yourself that you can and will appear confident. Most public icons, film stars, use their "fuel" to look confident, but as we see in news and tabloids, they are not. Even a simple smile shows confidence and appeal. In fact, the starting point to exuding your power starts with confidence.

Own your body image. If you're dissatisfied with your body, by all means, work on getting healthier, but remember that "sexy" or "confidence" isn't a body shape. It's an aura. Getting slim and toned can augment sexiness, but it can never replace it. Owning a Steinway isn't the same thing as being a master pianist; in the same way, owning a "hot" body isn't the same thing as being sexy. Learn to play the "piano" you've got. Work it and love it and everyone else will too.

Highlight your positive features. If you have pretty-blue-eyes, then show them off. If you have a beautiful smile, then flash those pearly whites. From beautiful eyes to statement jewelry or even makeup, may make a difference for you. Be classy. You're classy. Try to maintain class as much as possible while still being sexy.

Wear pretty lingerie and underwear, even if no one sees it. Pick some clothes that flatter your figure and that you feel comfortable in. There's no point picking the latest fashions if you don't feel comfortable in them. Invest in a good pair of curve-hugging jeans. Dark denim looks good on all body types. Black is sexy. It hides and creates curves and makes you feel like a goddess.

Take up dancing. Sign up for dance lessons with a friend, salsa, ballet, hip-hop, belly dancing, ballroom, whatever you like. Dancing is a wonderful way to learn who you are and find out what makes you feel sexy and confident. You'll gain confidence, and you will move more gracefully and sensual in everything you do, without even thinking about it. Health benefits are an obvious bonus.

Find your passion in life. Most of us are perceived much more confident when we find and live our passion in life. You come across knowledgeable, confident, strong, and energized. Your passion is turned into "FUEL".

This could be very uncomfortable, or it can be fun and exciting. But you must take the first step. Let go of resistance and any fear of change. Whether it be, change in your personality, dress, or favorite place to hang out. Once you decide that, you should be able to embrace your internal fuel, get comfortable IN it. That confidence and self-awareness can indeed alter how you are perceived by using your strong source of fuel.

How we use our fuel determines our level of mindfulness. Are you able to stay present and purposeful when it comes to steps you need to take in order to live your best sex life? Are you able to adjust and free your mind and allow yourself to be still? Take all the things off your mind and learn to just be. When you are still, you connect with breath and breath is very important when it comes to achieving orgasm and aiding in the intensity.

Of course, mindfulness is the new buzz word but don't let that scare you. It truly has been proven to manifest change through its use. It takes work to make it a habit so take baby steps, but work on things that will get you closer to the practice of mindfulness. It will make a difference in your intimate relationships. It will make a difference when it comes to your orgasm. So, I must share how to prepare your mind for an orgasm.

HOW TO RELAX

When you find yourself preparing for sex, you may find that you go into the experience much more relax than you may be used to. Foremost remember that YOU CANNOT have an orgasm if you are not completely relaxed, aroused and present. This could all mean different things to you. If you are going into sexual experiences to receive the benefits of the blood rush and increased oxygen you need to relax and breath through orgasm.

Relax — Resist Tension — Relax Deeper

Allow the muscles in your body to move rhythmically, only tensing to move. Any muscle not involved in motion should be relaxed and open. Your natural urge will be to tense with pleasure. Resist this urge and relax more deeply. Every muscle not being used in the present moment should be completely at rest.

Be Present

Remember to stay in the present, and not go off into your mind, or into thoughts about what is coming next, or what just happened, or what may or may not happen. Notice what is going on inside you and through you in the present moment and stay with that. This is like being "in the zone" while performing music, playing sports, or engaging in improvisational comedy. Stay in the zone. Don't allow your awareness to drift off somewhere else. Staying present to what you are sensing in the body and feeling in the emotions. Notice how it changes and shifts from one moment to the next, and ride the wave higher and higher, like a surfer on the biggest and best ride of a lifetime.

UNDERSTANDING ORGASM

Orgasms, been around since the dawn of time, right? You would be surprised. The orgasm has been around but was believed to be the result of sexual stimulation in men only. Its definition read: a climax of sexual excitement, characterized by feelings of pleasure centered in the genitals and (in men) experienced as an accompaniment to ejaculation. As if to say that one could not happen without the other but more disturbing that the female had no such pleasure, especially anything that was an accompaniment to ejaculation!

It was not until the late 1950s that research showed that the female body did have physical reactions to sexual stimulation. That the internal genitals of the female also could swell and have reactions similar to that of a man. Even EJACULATE! This, my friends, is the mental block we women have been birthed into. The mindset hadn't changed from a time when women who squirted used to be burned at the stake. We now know that this is a very normal, globally achieved reaction to stimulation. It's the mental drilling of mixed messages about any pleasure received during sex.

What we learn to do always only leads to the Genital Orgasm. A Genital Orgasm is quite easy to achieve by comparison to a Deep Orgasm. We see the techniques that lead to Genital Orgasm demonstrated in movies, in pornography, and in our comedic representations of sex. Whether a person has ever had an orgasm, most people at least understand some of the ways to achieve a Genital Orgasm, simply from watching popular media or from their friends.

ORGASM PROCESS

Research shows that what happens in a woman's body during orgasm involves many parts of the female anatomy. Depending on the intensity of the orgasm, the vagina, uterus, anus, hands, feet, and abdomen contract rapidly. 3–15 times, squeezing for 0.8 seconds at a time (Rimm, H., December 11, 2017). When women ejaculate, the fluid released comes from the urethra, as we stated, and emits a clear/whitish fluid from the urethra opening. This is why it feels like pee; it shares the urethra tube and is near the bladder causing the pressure feeling. When you feel this, breath in deeply and allow the orgasm to wash over you. If you are an orgasmic individual, you will ejaculate.

STAGES OF ORGASM

Getting a handle on your understanding or orgasms can help you achieve them. Arm yourself with as much information as possible. The sexual response cycle includes four stages (Rimm, H., December 11, 2017).

Excitement: Initially being turned on.

Plateau: Repetitive motion that feels pleasurable.

Orgasm: The burst of pleasure, and release.

Resolution: The refractory period.

You should know that these stages are subjective. Things to consider are the size of the orgasm, which could range differently for everyone. Someone's experience won't be your experience, so don't set yourself up for failure by trying to reach their experience. Also, bodies are different. The path that your body needs to get to orgasm is going to be based on your experimenting, communication, and practicing.

Let's say we are at the point where you believe you can't orgasm. This is when you want to call in someone like me to help you overcome barriers to your orgasm. The issue could be as simple as switching your medication or increasing the strength of your pelvic floor.

We'll discuss the multiple phases of orgasm and their benefits to the female body.

TENSION & RELAXATION

Around 10% of women have never had an orgasm via with a partner or masturbation (Weston, 2018). This could be for several reasons; however, you can learn to be orgasmic.

To begin, practice developing a balance of tension and relaxation during sexual activity. This is the internal battle our bodies put us through during orgasm. This is why it may be so hard to achieve. Your natural instinct is to hold your breath through pleasure, yet if you breathed and relaxed, you would build up an orgasm and with practice, they can become more and more intense.

Weston gives two of the tips she uses with her clients to bring about orgasms (Weston, 2018), that I have seen work quite well. The first is a dedication to strengthen your pelvic floor muscles. This comes from Step 1: Tense Up.

The type of tension that helps women reach orgasm is muscle tension. Women believe that they just need to relax and lay there and wait for an orgasm. It is true that relaxation is also needed in this step. Of course, it is. You cannot stay in a state of tension for an extended period of time. This is the balance you must learn, between tension and relaxing. The tension in the muscles are good for an orgasm. Incorporating an amount of leg, abdominal, and buttock tension all aid in reaching an orgasm.

Research has determined that orgasm-inducing muscle contractions are in the lower pelvis during the peak. We know that these are the same muscles you squeeze to stop the flow of urine. The official name for this exercise is a Kegel, named after the doctor that discovered the benefits of this technique. (Weston, 2018)

The thing that connects the tensing muscle groups to the orgasm is arousal. The contractions cause an increase in blood flow throughout the body and most beneficially, the genitals. Most vulva born females cannot reach orgasm without being aroused. This is why keeping an arsenal of foreplay strategies in your repertoire is a plus.

Step 2. Wind Down. This is the relaxation part of the exercise. It's winding down the brain and focusing in on things that are happening to bring on the orgasm. During sex, focus simply on feeling the sensations of the stimulation (Weston, 2018).

Weston shares a tip to keep you focus on the moment and not your to-do list. She says, "think of a Times Square billboard in which words stream into view from the left-hand side to the right edge, and then disappear off the screen. During sex, many women find it helpful to program their own Times Square news crawl with a repetitive mantra such as "I can take as long as I want" or "This really feels great" on their mental silent radio. It keeps the brain occupied, but with a thought that will encourage sexual arousal rather than with a nervous, negative thought that might decrease arousal" (Weston, 2018).

We can all try this technique and tense up our pelvic floors, use our abs muscles. Squeeze as if you are holding in gas and stopping the flow of urine. Try and concentrate on the tension and finding pleasure. From any source, a sexy memory maybe. When you can no longer hold that tension, take a sigh of release. Notice that flutter of pleasure your body experiences as you allow it to receive air again. This is the process of building arousal. Continue to tense up the muscles and let the mind go silent. This takes a ton of practice. If you are committed to having orgasms or increasing the intensity of your orgasm, then learning the balance between tension and relaxation is the exercise to commit to.

ENJOY STRONGER ORGASMS

There are many types of orgasms, but for the purposes of this discussion, we'll be grouping them into two broad categories: *The Genital Orgasm* and *The Deep Orgasm*. How you feel about your partner has a great deal to do with it. If you're involving yourself in purely casual relationships, it may be more difficult to achieve. If you're diving in deep to truly intimate and authentic relating, then it may be much easier to achieve.

A Genital / Clitoral focused orgasm, which is very pleasurable, focused primarily in the lower regions in or near the genitals, sometimes includes more "full body" effects such as shaking or shuddering body, sometimes is accompanied by involuntary noise-making, and is rarely ejaculatory.

A Deep / Full-Body orgasm, which is usually substantially more pleasurable (women report to be between 2 times and 100 times more powerful than the Genital Orgasm), focused throughout the entire body, almost always includes more "full body" effects such as shaking or shuddering body, almost always is accompanied by involuntary noise-making, and is often potentially ejaculatory.

The Deep Orgasm is mysterious to many. People spend years seeking the experience, and the problem is that the way to reach one is counter intuitive. It requires a kind of impulse-denying mechanism to reach one. Many of the things the human body naturally seems to want to do during sex, and many of our most common human psychological blocks, actually get directly in the way of achieving this type of orgasm

How to Achieve Genital Orgasm

Most penis owners have figured out how to have this type of orgasm through masturbation, so my advice will mainly be targeted at pre-orgasmic vulva owners. The same techniques, however, may be used by all to achieve similar results.

Breathe: Remember to breathe while engaged in sexual activity, including while masturbating. There is a natural tendency to hold the breath at the end of an inhale while masturbating, and sometimes also at the end of an exhale. Allow the breath to be continuous. When the breath fills the lungs, do not stop, continue to exhale immediately, and when the breath empties the lungs, do not stop, continue to inhale immediately. Always keep the breath moving.

Make Sounds: Sound will always help you have a deeper and more powerful sexual experience, whether you're looking for an orgasm or just pleasure, and regardless of the type of orgasm you want. This one tends to be most difficult for people, of all the advice I'm going to offer here. People are self-conscious about how they sound, and even worse, afraid someone will hear them when masturbating. Learn to be okay with your sounds and to express them fully. Make the sound of how you feel in the moment, as distinct from a performance sound This is not about turning them on — it is about expressing how you are feeling in your body and emotions in the moment.

Feel Yourself: Be both physically and emotionally present to what you are feeling. What does that touch feel like? What would that feel like somewhere else? Where in your body are your emotions and what are they doing in the present moment?

Be Present: If you are alone and fantasizing, be present to yourself, to your emotions, to your sensations, to your sounds, and your fantasy. If you are with a partner, throw out any fantasies and be present to your partner. Gaze into their eyes. Permit yourself to look at whatever you want. Be present to what you want in the moment and go for it.

Tense Before the Orgasmic Wave: When you feel yourself building toward a peak of pleasure, tense the muscles in your core: the buttocks, abdominals, and thighs. Inhale deeply and briefly hold your breath, only for a few seconds. On the exhale, release all the tension and allow the orgasm to come over you. You may need to repeat this step a few times, depending on how "high" your wave is, and how much "pressure" is built up behind the wave.

If you follow these techniques, even if does not happen the first time, it is likely you will soon reach orgasm.

One of the most important parts is to become comfortable with yourself, your sexual sensations and emotions, and your expression of your sexuality. Give yourself permission for it to show up however it shows up. There is no right or wrong way to sexual pleasure. Allow yourself total freedom in expressing the way you feel and doing what you want to do.

Release and Relax into the Orgasmic Wave: Unlike the genital orgasm, you want to avoid tension as much as possible. For some vulva owners (generally not for penis owners) it may be useful to bear down at the last moment before the deep orgasm as if you were attempting to urinate. First, try this orgasm without any bearing down, and see what happens. Relax completely. It will be natural to feel an urge to tense up when you near orgasm. Resist this urge, and instead relax fully and completely. Surrender to the orgasm. Let go. Let every muscle go and allow the deep orgasm to wash over you and through you. This may feel like "too much." The experience is very intense, and the amount of emotion and sensation is literally off-the-charts when compared to a genital orgasm.

It only feels like "too much" because you're not used to it yet. Relax, breathe, soften the muscles and the movements. Soften the face and the voice. Let go. Surrender. Experience true bliss. You may feel as if you're about to urinate. This is not urination. This is ejaculation. If you have never experienced it before, ejaculation may feel the same as urination, but it is NOT pee. If you have experienced ejaculation before, you will always know the difference between how the ejaculation feels and how urination feels. You do not need to stop to urinate; the PC muscle controls which fluid is released. The hormones tell the PC muscle, and it happens automatically, just like in penis born individuals.

Keep going. Relax. Let go. Surrender. Allow yourself to ejaculate. Let go and surrender to the power of orgasm.

How to Achieve Deep Orgasm: This is the type of orgasm that remains shrouded in mystery for most people, even after many thousands of years our species has lived on this planet. It is precisely because a lot of the advice I am going to give is counter-intuitive and because the genital orgasm is so much simpler and more intuitive to achieve that the deep orgasm has remained shrouded in mystery. I aim to dispel that mystery and break down the deep orgasm into some simple instructions that anyone can follow.

When attempting this type of orgasm, my advice is to take 4-8 bath towels and fold them in half (so they're squares, rather than rectangular), and place them under you. This is a precaution, as you are much more likely to ejaculate during this type of orgasm, and the towels make it "okay" to "wet the bed." The towels serve as a kind of permission slip to let go.

To create a Deep Orgasm, prepare your partner by utilizing all of the erogenous zones to arouse them to ecstasy. Begin with the softer subtle areas. Use your tongue, teeth, lips, fingers and toes to caress and massage to relax your mate and prepare them for more intense pleasure. Based on the positive reaction you get, move on to include the genitals. Slowly caressing the lips, using the moisture that is there to make the area slick. This will add pleasure to the strokes. Continue to build up their orgasms by staying connected with their body and making confident moves. If finger play is the next phase, use one of the three finger techniques to stimulate the G Spot, the A spot deep spot and the C spot. Stimulation to these areas will bring on intense orgasms. Each feeling different than the other. Proceed to penetration of preference and bring attention to the clitoris until your mate is having a mind-blowing orgasm. Be sure to stay with them to the end of the orgasm, don't stop short, ride the wave with them. It's rare but possible to orgasm together.

How Do You Tell the Difference Between These Orgasms? Once you have had both, you'll know the difference every time, but here are a few indicators:

- How long did the peak of pleasure last? If only 10 seconds to 30 seconds, you probably had a genital orgasm. If 30 seconds to 5 minutes, you probably had a deep orgasm.

- How many waves did the orgasm have? If only one, you may have had a genital orgasm. If two or more, you may have had a deep orgasm.

- Did the orgasm feel "typical" to you? If so, you probably had a genital orgasm. If it felt two times greater than "typical" or more than that, then you may have had a deep orgasm.

- If you own a penis, did you ejaculate? If yes, you probably had a genital orgasm. If no, you probably had a deep orgasm.

- If you're a vulva owner did you ejaculate? If yes, you probably had a deep orgasm. If no, you probably had a genital orgasm.

A Technique for Pre-Orgasmic Vulva Owners: If you or your partner are pre-orgasmic, you may wish to try this technique of pleasuring in order to bring them to their first orgasm. First, you must learn what gives them the most pleasure. Hopefully, they have explored themselves enough to know the answer to this question, but if not, you'll need to explore their body using your hands, tongue, penis, and any other body parts that seem appropriate. Find out what gives them the most pleasure.

Second, tell them that as you provide pleasure in this way that she most enjoys, she must relax completely. Say that if you feel them tense up, you will stop what you are doing and tease them until their pleasure subsides a bit.

Follow through on this promise. Because it is natural to tense the body during pleasure, they will no-doubt tense up. Each time the muscles tense up, back off from their most pleasurable areas and techniques, and tease them until their breathing slows and they relax again, and remind them gently, "you tensed up, so I'm going to tease you now." Third, tell them to always breathe. Say that if you feel them stop breathing, you will tease them until their pleasure subsides. Pay attention to the breath, and when they stop breathing, another natural response during sexual pleasure, follow through on your promise. Gently remind them, "you forgot to breathe, so

I'm going to tease you." Tease mercilessly until they calm down and backs off from the pleasurable peak.

Continue the above, and repeat, repeat, repeat again. Repeat again and again until they say something like this, and you know it to be very authentically self-expressed: "PLEASE, DON'T STOP!" Really wait for them to beg for you not to stop.

Erogenous Zones

P arts of the vulva, especially the clitoris, are erogenous zones. While the vagina is not especially sensitive as a whole, its lower third (the area close to the entrance) has concentrations of the nerve endings that can provide pleasurable sensations during sexual activity when stimulated; this is also called the anterior wall of the vagina or the outer one-third of the vagina, and it contains the majority of the vaginal nerve endings, making it more sensitive to touch than the inner two-thirds of the vaginal barrel.

Within the anterior wall of the vagina, there is a patch of ribbed rough tissue which has a texture that is sometimes described as similar to the palate (the roof of a mouth) or a raspberry and may feel spongy when a vulva owner is sexually aroused. This is the urethral sponge, which may also be the location of the G-spot — a structure described as an area of the vagina that some women report is an erogenous zone which, when stimulated, can lead to sexual arousal, orgasms, and ejaculation. The existence of the G-spot and whether or not it is a distinct structure is debated among researchers; as reports of its location vary from vulva to vulva, it appears to be nonexistent in some, and scientists commonly believe that it is an extension of the clitoris.

Vulva owners are equipped with the ability to have different types of orgasms with a variety of feelings and levels of intensity associated with them. They are "built" with the capacity to reach orgasms of different types.

YONI MASSAGE

Most may call the act of a stranger stroking or rubbing (NEVER orally) an intimate and relaxing experience. Yes, people are paying experts, usually a Professional Tantric Practitioner, to "massage" your vagina. Yoni, named after the Sanskrit word for vagina, is much like other massages. It too is designed to release tension. The yoni is one of the most intimate and powerful parts of the body it's important that the massage follows certain guidelines — a ritual sort of. Yoni massage is profound work. A Tantric tradition studied deeply and thoroughly. Professional practitioners should have years of experience and have studied with reputable organizations. A person interested in yoni massage should get a recommendation from someone who has received one firsthand. Do not go blindly into a consultation. It should be stated that most clients will or may have a clitoral orgasm during or at the end of the massage. This is simply part of the experience; it is not followed by further stimulation or sexual intercourse.

CLITORAL ORGASM

When stimulated, 8,000 nerve fibers of the clitoris interact with 15,000 nerve fibers in the pelvic area, leading to an intense orgasm. There are 18 parts to the clitoris, inside and outside of the body. The clitoris is a sex pleasure piece of heaven on earth. It is the most sensitive spot on the ENTIRE body.

It is well known as the hot spot. It is located at the top of the vulva. Right where the inner labia join the upper ends. The visible part is the small, nipple size sensitive item. It is the vulva equivalent of the tip of the penis. The clit is often hidden by a protective hood. It has purely a sexual function; it enlarges (erect) making it even more sensitive. During foreplay, it is often stimulated directly by touch, and many do not easily reach orgasm purely from vaginal stimulation find it easier to climax from oral, digital, or mechanical stimulation of the clitoris.

The most interesting part of the history of studying the female body, it was said that women did not have orgasms or a need to enjoy sex. The purpose of sex was to procreate. It should be stated that most studies were conduct and analyzed by men. Due to continued research, we now know that the clitoris is larger than first reported. Most of it is hidden within the vagina.

The part we do see is literally just the tip. Within the walls or shaft, it extends down to surround the vaginal opening. Thus, during pelvic thrusting, the part you can't see will be massaged vigorously by the movements of insertion. Doing so will provide clitoral stimulation. Some folks claim that, by employing a rhythmic, downward roll of the pelvis, they can create a direct friction on the clitoris tip while the mate is making pelvic thrusts and can in this way magnify their arousal. This requires a more dominant role for the receiver. It is also known that clitoral orgasms can be extended. By extended, I mean 20 seconds to a few moments. They are very deep clitoral orgasms and surface clitoral orgasms.

Stimulating the clitoris and pressure in or around the vagina can cause pelvic fullness and body tension to build up to a peak. During sexual excitement, the clitoris swells and changes position. The blood vessels through the whole pelvic area also swell, causing engorgement and a feeling of fullness and sexual sensitivity.

You or a partner can stimulate your clitoris in a few different ways — by rubbing, sucking, body pressure, or using a vibrator. Although some women touch the glans of the clitoris to become aroused, for others, it can be so sensitive that direct touching hurts, even with lubrication. Also, focusing directly on the clitoris for a long time may cause the pleasurable sensations to disappear. Your clitoris can also be stimulated during sexual intercourse, most often with you on top — this happens when the clitoris is rubbed against the mate's pubic bone.

It can also be achieved when the giver is on top and if they position themselves high enough so that the pubic bone presses against your clitoral area. The simple fact is, you or your partner can also stimulate your clitoris with fingers during intercourse to help bring you to orgasm.

VAGINAL ORGASM

A "vaginal orgasm" is the notion that vagina born individuals can have an orgasm through stimulation during intercourse or other vaginal penetration, entirely without clitoral stimulation. Only 25% of vulva born individuals can achieve orgasm during thrusting. Why? Those who have a shorter distance between their clitoris and their urethral mentus can better reach an orgasm this way because the clitoris is indirectly stimulated during sex. For the other 75%, it is difficult to achieve the 'O' this way.

Research conducted by a female scientist determined that the vaginal canal has few nerve endings, and therefore may not create an orgasm on its own. There is not a total separation between the vagina and clitoris; most think this is based on a misunderstanding of what, where, and how big the clitoris really is.

A group of 27 couples were asked to vary their sexual positions experimentally, employing postures that would allow greater stimulation of the two vaginal 'hot spots,' and it was found that three-quarters of the females involved were then able to achieve regular vaginal orgasms.

A "vaginal orgasm" is the notion that folks can have an orgasm through stimulation during intercourse or other vaginal penetration, entirely without clitoral stimulation.

The clitoral organ system actually surrounds the vagina, urethra, and anus. Rather than thinking of an orgasm as "vaginal" or "clitoral", it makes more sense to think of orgasm in terms of the feelings that came along with it. The emphasis on stimulation from penetration makes the folic/fingers central to sexual satisfaction.

It is important to emphasize again that these statements were not based on a study of women's anatomy, but rather upon assumptions of women as inferior to men. The inner vaginal lips swell and change shape, and the vagina balloons upward, causing the uterus to shift position.

Orgasm is the point at which all the tension is suddenly released in a series of involuntary and pleasurable muscular contractions in the vagina, uterus, and/or rectum.

A-SPOT

This is the anterior fornix erogenous zone of the vagina, where it is more sensitive to touch than the inner two-thirds of the vaginal canal. A patch of sensitive tissue at the inner end of the vaginal tube between the cervix and the bladder described technically as the 'female degenerated prostate'. It may feel spongy when aroused, which is why it is also called the urethral sponge. This orgasm is achieved by stimulating about 3-4 inches deep in the top wall of the vagina.

Many have never heard of the A spot and are missing out on a major source of pleasure. There are two positions that work best, missionary and the cowgirl. In the missionary position, place pillows under their back to provide the best angle for penetration. In cowgirl, the receiver is on top of the giver facing them. Have them lean back a little so a dildo/penis can thrust deeper inside to reach past the G-spot.

One of the main reasons why it is easier for them to have multiple orgasms with the A-spot is that it does not become overly sensitive like the clitoris can. Many can have two or more orgasms via deeper penetration and A-spot massage Direct stimulation of this spot can produce violent orgasmic contractions. Unlike the clitoris, it is not supposed to suffer from post-orgasmic over-sensitivity. Its existence was reported by a Malaysian physician in Kuala Lumpur as recently as the 1990s. The uterus's cervix is the narrow part that protrudes slightly into the vagina, leaving a circular recess around itself. Pressure on it produces rapid lubrication of the vagina, even for those who are not normally sexually responsive.

It is now possible to buy a special AFE vibrator — long thin and upward curved at its end, to probe this zone. It has been claimed that two out of every three participants fail to reach regular orgasms from simple penetrative sex.

DEEP SPOT ORGASM

This orgasm can be achieved by stimulating the deepest back wall of the vagina right behind the cervix. It may be difficult to reach the spot without causing initial discomfort. (some hate to have the cervix touched) It can also deliver THE most INTENSE and POWERFUL ORGASM. Typically, a vibrator is used to stimulate the deep spot. You can also use 2 fingers, be gentle but purposeful. DO NOT push pass anything that feels "unforgiving". Meaning anything firm or solid. This note is IMPORTANT for all vaginal play.

You'll feel the cervix as a small hole; the deep spot orgasm can be found behind the cervix all the way to the back of the vagina in a bunny hop motion with your fingers move up and down. Having your mate raise their knees to their chest intensifies this deep orgasm because it is also manipulating the skene's gland (female prostate) at the same time and may cause multiple orgasms.

Your partner should lie on her back and spread her legs with her knees bent. Put a lot of lubricant on your fingers and be careful not to damage the inside of her vagina with your fingernails. Slide your middle finger up the upper wall of the vagina deep inside her, with your palm facing upward. You'll first feel the rough part, where the G-spot is also situated, then the smooth and slippery part, where you can also feel the cervix. Curl your fingertip into the 'bunny hop' position and press firmly against the back wall of the vagina. Start massaging the deep spot firmly as if you were thrusting with your fingers. Be careful that your hand is moist enough with the lubricant and that the massage is firm. Your fingertip should literally become immersed into the soft walls of her vagina.

U-SPOT ORGASM

This orgasm can be achieved by stimulating a small area that contains sensitive erectile tissue located directly above and on either side of the urethra opening. It sits in the small area between the urethra and the vagina opening. The American Clinical research team found that the U-spot, when gently caressed, with the finger, the tongue, or folic, gave powerful erotic response.

Your partner should lie on their back with her legs relaxed. If needed, gently use your forearms to aid in keeping them open and spread the labia's. Again, as always, unless you are told otherwise, be gentle. Push ever so slight up on the clitoris hood and 1 of several things should happen: pushing back the space opened a small area between the valley peak of labia and clitoris, the clitoris swells and extends toward you, creating about a pinky nail size space that is tender, yet firm, or nothing.

The second three happens stop and try another method. Both of these incidents would not allow this particular individual to orgasm and it's a nice trick to share with your friends. If either of the first two, use a sensitive, soft, almost ticklish tongue to long stroke the length and width of this space. It may take several minutes to reach the point of orgasm for most of us. Try a few of these tricks to learn what works for this person.

- A quick light/medium/hard, flickering tip of tongue

- A soft puckering(kiss), popping.

- Alterations in firm/fast, firm/soft, soft/wet, firm/wet

Note: Noise may or may not be controllable.

BREAST ORGASM

Some vulva born individuals can reach orgasm by the stimulus of their breasts if present. This is an orgasm that comes from sudden discharge of sexual tension while manipulated. The stimulation leads to the expansion of the breast releasing oxytocin that leads to release. The feeling of radiating sensations around the breast, a fullness and nipple erection of the tissue can drive a person to orgasm. Massaging, squeezing, pinching, licking, and biting are all actions that can get them there.

Most vulva born individuals get aroused by having their nipples touched, and this may or may not lead to an orgasm. Let your partner know what you like and don't like about your breast stimulation. The size of the breast does not matter. It has been proven that larger breasts are more sensitive. The size of the nipples doesn't count either. What matters is the fact that breast may be more sensitive before, during, or after the menstrual cycle. There is less sensitivity or greater sensitivity during ovulation and lessened sensitivity during menses. A breast orgasm is a little different than vaginal orgasms. Some people note contractions in the uterus that they don't feel during clitoral stimulation. For some, they don't feel a connection between the breast and genital stimulation opposite having the genitals stimulated.

What gives rise to a breast orgasm?

It has been described by various doctors as an occurrence that happens at the peak of sexual stimulation where the sensation seems to be radiating from around the breast area. It is claimed to be the second most common orgasm among women. The nipples are the main players when it comes to breast orgasms. They are filled with nerve endings making them very sensitive to touch. Also, it is important to note that researchers discovered that the stimulation of the nipple activated an area of the brain known as the genital sensory cortex. It is the same area that is activated by stimulation of the clitoris, cervix, and vagina.

Bottom Line

As not every individual gets breast orgasms, there is a way in which the orgasms may be brought to life. This happens when the correct nerve impulses relate to the correct moves. It is important to note that a s partner should be able to prepare them well before beginning to stimulate their breasts. Kissing and teasing their nipples first would do the trick. Sucking of the nipples should follow, but the partner should make sure that they are not being rough or aggressive as this may irritate the person. It is also important to realize that it is basically the tongue that does all the work as it drives them to orgasmic pleasure. It may take quite some time before you get the orgasm, but all the time and effort will definitely be worth it.

ORAL ORGASM

Some are very sensitive in their mouths and can reach orgasm when kissing or receiving/performing oral sex.

There are so many ways to express your love, but none so tender as the kiss. Come and deepen your intimacy and bring more fun and playfulness into your relationship. The kiss is more than just a powerful form of foreplay.

When you kiss someone, you are saying in every molecule of your body that which cannot be conveyed with words. The kiss is one of the holiest things that can be exchanged between two people. This is your holy grail, and you are allowing another to drink from your sacred cup. Kissing is a most powerful way for couples to express their devotion, tenderness and fully surrender to the passion of the moment.

SKIN ORGASM

Some folks can reach orgasm at the touch of their skin, during a massage, a facial, or any stimulus to their skin. Perhaps most often while listening to music. You may feel a fluttering in your stomach, a shiver down your spine and a racing heart when they listen to music. The aesthetic experience can be so intense that you can't do anything else. However, the tendency for classical music to be the main cause of these reactions may be more due to bias in research than anything unique about it.

Researchers say other music genres like pop, folk and those from elsewhere in the world could also trigger similar responses. There are several theories that are thought to explain why the human body reacts in this way to music. It is thought that it is linked to the release of dopamine in the brain — a hormone that deals with emotion and reward. The auditory area is also thought to be connected to the emotional and reward processing areas of the brain. Another study found that around 24% of people experience tears, 10% get shivers, while 5% get goosebumps on their skin.

Music is well known for its power to move listeners, often to tears, but there are some people who experience it so intensely they compare it to having an orgasm.

The sensation, known as a skin orgasms, produces a feeling of pleasure so intense it can be felt all over their body, can produce trembling, sweating and even arousal. A team of researchers has highlighted the powerful reaction in a recent review of the evidence surrounding people's physical response to music.

MENTAL ORGASM

Some people can reach orgasm during auditory or visual stimulation, like watching a movie, reading, erotic content, or watching others having sex. This orgasm happens without manual or oral stimulations. The technique can also be used by people with sexual dysfunction, those who have had clitorectomies, and anyone with a physical condition that makes genital orgasms difficult or impossible.

Mind-blowing orgasms can be had through breath and energy. This kind of orgasm requires you to create energy between you. Mental orgasms can be powerful. Those who can experience them describe them as being an all-over body pleasure. Some intense orgasms such as this one, have led people to nervous breakdowns and paralysis. Breath and energy orgasms can occur from conscious, rhythmic, deep breathing, or other ways of generating energy in the body such as swimming, running, risk taking, listening to a piece of music, etc.

The brain is the most powerful sex organ. It is heavily involved in the orgasm process. Sex is defined by our senses, perceptions, and memories. Mental stimulation can get an orgasm started. Relaxing and enjoying the sensations instead of thinking of other things allows the orgasm to build and be released.

G-SPOT ORGASM

Named after Dr. Ernst Gräfenberg who first wrote about it in 1950, crazy right, it is a sensitive area located just behind the frontal wall of the vulva, right within the first 2-3 inches of the vaginal canal. It is not a button; it is an area that is located between the clitoral legs that are internal. The G-spot is an erogenous zone that can lead to arousal into an ejaculatory orgasm.

This is a form of orgasm that will cause them to squirt. This differs from vaginal lubrication, in fact, carried out by the walls of the vagina which rapidly becomes covered in a liquid film when sexual arousal first begins. There are specialized glands surrounding the urethral tube, called Skene's glands, or para-urethral glands, similar to the prostate, and under extreme stimulation, they produce an alkaline liquid that is chemically similar to seminal fluid. If you can experience ejaculation, it will range in quantity from two teaspoons to cups full. Some imagine that the extreme muscular exertions of their climactic moments have forced them into involuntary urination, but this is simply because they do not understand their own physiology.

Penis born individuals deliver sperm and urine through the urethral tube and it was believed that only urine passes through the vagina born individual. Research shows that this is not the case; when there is powerful enough orgasm, they can release fluid from their urethral opening that is not urine. As mentioned before, this is because of the Skene's glands that surround both sides of the urethral. They can release anywhere between a few tablespoons to cups of a clear, odorless fluid known as squirting.

I hold a G-spot workshop at most of my larger parties and for expos such as Sexaplooza and eXXXOtica. I have seen this happen for women who claim they don't have orgasms, let alone could bring forth ejaculate. This is a small, highly sensitive area located 5-8 cm (2-3 inches) inside the vagina, on the front or upper wall. Research into the nature of the vulva owner orgasm, carried out in the 1940s, led to the discovery that the urethral tube that lies on top of the vagina is surrounded by erectile tissue similar to that found in the penis.

When the person becomes sexually aroused, this tissue starts to swell. In the G-spot zone, this expansion resides in a small patch of the vaginal wall protruding into the vaginal canal. A primary erotic zone, perhaps more important than the clitoris. The significance was lost when the 'missionary position' became a dominant feature of human sexual behavior. Other sexual positions are far more efficient at stimulating this erogenous zone and, therefore, achieving an ejaculate orgasm.

Some women have been led to believe, optimistically, that there is a 'sex button' that can be pressed like a starter button, at any time, to cause an erotic explosion. Disappointed, they then conclude that the whole concept of a 'G-spot' is false and that it does not exist. As already explained, the truth is that the G-spot is a sexually sensitive patch of vaginal wall that protrudes slightly only when the glands surrounding the urethral tube have become swollen.

Several leading gynecologists denied its existence when it was first discussed at their conferences, and a major controversy arose, but later, when it was specially demonstrated for their benefit, they changed their minds. Sexual politics also entered the debate when certain anti-male campaigners rejected out of hand the idea that vaginal orgasm could be possible.

For them, clitoral orgasm was politically correct, and no other would do. How they have reacted to the recent marketing of 'G-spotter' attachments for vibrators is not recorded. Astonishingly, there have been recent reports that some people have been undergoing 'G-spot enhancement.' This involves injecting collagen into the G-spot zone to enlarge it. According to one source, one of the latest procedures to catch on is G-spot injection. Similar substances to those injected into the lips to plump them up can now be injected into your G-spot. The idea is that this will increase its sensitivity and so give you better orgasms.

MEGAGASM

These are the volcano of all orgasms, or the tsunami of all orgasms. A megagasm is an intense full body experience, a deeply emotional experience, and for some, a deeply spiritual experience. It lasts an extended lengthy of time, from thirty seconds to, in some cases, up to an hour or two.

Several megagasm have been documented on video, although they are extremely rare. Not that many vulva owners are capable of letting go that deeply or handling that much pleasure and ecstasy and orgasmic energy. Megagasm are usually brought about by very intense physical stimulation—with very hard fucking combined with a really strong vibrator on the clitoris, fist fucking, anal sex with vaginal and clitoral stimulation, etc. Sometimes some discomfort or pain can trigger one.

The stimulation goes way beyond normal lovemaking, into surrendering to intense physical force and massive genital manipulation. It helps to have an 'orgasm midwife', someone who is totally present that can manage and handle the incredible intensity of such orgasms. Many people can be very scared of and uncomfortable with the force of megagasm. The person having the orgasm's face can severely contort like one is having a baby; there is a huge ego surrender.

Megagasm can come with past life recalls and intense visual imagery like with psychedelics. It can feel as if there is a lifetime of pent up energy and emotion bursting free. They are very primal. There can be a sensation of being 'breathed by the universe', like you are a channel for orgasmic energy like you are open for the life force to pass through you. Often people will have empathetic orgasms when they are in the presence of someone having megagasm.

As an orgasm coach, I strive to help all my clients get to their best orgasm. Orgasm is not always the wanted result; however, if you are one who embraces the orgasm and all its pleasure, you should refer back to this section often. This is what you are looking for. If you have never experienced an orgasm, be sure you are not overlooking the signs that you are building and pay attention to the feelings and react freely.

If you do not reach the type of orgasm you're seeking the first time, keep practicing. It is not always easy to reach orgasm, especially deep orgasm, and especially for vulva owners. Don't make yourself wrong for failing. Keep practicing. You will get there. In either case, failure in the moment is not failure forever. Keep taking it to new heights. Keep surrendering to pleasure. You will arrive at your destination if you remember to breathe, to relax, and to surrender to your feelings in the present.

Bigger Bodied Sex

B igger bodied individuals have amazing sex all the time. However, size can sometimes cause certain positions not to work so well. Here are some of the best positions for bigger individuals and how you can modify sex positions to work even though you may be big and beautiful. These positions are for individuals having penetrative sex. I will refer to the folic having mate as the "giver" and will use "receiver" for the mate being penetrated. You may find that memory foam pillows become your best buddy.

Take the worry of what your mate may think of your body off the table. They might specifically like how you look and feel because you're fluffier. I tell people to have sex with the lights on at least some of the time because confidence is very sexy! You should do your best to focus on how sex feels and not how it looks. Even the most gorgeous people can get into unflattering positions, but you know why they do that? Because it feels good for them or their partners! If you're constantly worried about how you look or sound during sex, you're unlikely to loosen up enough to an orgasm.

You might worry that you're not sure what to do. Being on top can look like it needs a lot of flexibility or strength, especially in porn, but that's not always the case. You don't necessarily have to rest on your feet and bounce. In fact, many receivers prefer kneeling and grinding back and forth, which can also provide better stimulation.

MODIFICATION IS KEY

Some of these positions need modification for rounded butts, bigger tummies, and more weight. A little modification goes a long way. You'll want to stay away from positions where you're facing each other.

This means things such as

- Kneeling rather than sitting or lying

- Moving to the floor instead of the soft bed

- Strategically placing pillows under the partner's body who is on the bottom

- Leaning over a piece of furniture

- Scooting to the end of the bed

- Lifting a leg

- Using your mates' shoulders

It's easy to think that sex should be, well, easy. But sometimes it takes a bit to figure out how best your bodies work together, and there's nothing wrong with that!

CAUSE FOR CONCERN

While being a bigger lover won't stop you from having a fun and active sex life if you don't let it, there are some considerations. For example, you don't want to get into any positions where your mate has to carry or hold you if they can't comfortably do that. Be sure to note weight limits on any sex furniture or sex swings or sinks. There are items made specifically for larger bodies. You don't want to come crashing down and hurt yourself.

POSITIONS WITH MODIFICATION

There are positions that don't have 'names" and some that are well known by many as known sexual positions. Here are a few that have modifications that will allow a bigger bodied individual to enjoy them all.

Doggy Style

Doggy style is a good position because your tummy can't get in the way. Instead, your giver enters you from behind. Rear entry positions can be more difficult if you've also got a bigger butt, however. Pillows, especially those made from memory foam, can help you support your weight in this position. Plus, doggy style is great for G-spot stimulation if that is a goal.

Cowgirl

The second position is one that many larger receivers are afraid to try. However, this position is ideal because your giver lies on the bed and you can straddle them and go to town. Fully controlling the depth and speed of the penetration. Plop a couple of pillows under the giver's butt to raise their hips for a better angle.

Spooning

This is another good sex position however, the folic needs to be long enough to penetrate you from behind. You are lying on your back. The giver can adjust their body, so they are at more of an angle than exactly parallel to your body. You are front to back. They can lean their top half away from you, potentially placing their legs between yours, so their feet stick out front and further extended the folic. Another option is for you to lift your leg, either bent at the knee or pointed toward the ceiling. This enables the giver to grab your leg for leverage and get closer to you for penetration.

Leg Glider

In the Leg Glider position, you're slightly leaning to one side (you can potentially lie on your back if you twist your spine, however). You lift your upper leg toward the ceiling, and the giver straddles your leg that is on the bed. They need to scoot close enough to penetrate, which means they can grasp your leg or place it along their body wherever your foot lands based on your height. This might be a good position for nuzzling, a leg massage or even some foot play if either of you has a foot kink. If your tummy prevents you from lifting your leg or get the most penetration, try lifting/shifting into a comfortable position.

Thigh Tide

Thigh Tide is just Reverse Cowgirl with an important alteration: the giver bends one leg at the knee, you can wrap your arms around their leg and grind your genitals against their thigh as you ride them. This increases the likelihood that you'll orgasm.

Butterfly

The final sex position works best if your mate is the right height to penetrate you while they stand on the floor and you lie on your back on the bed. In the Butterfly position, you should be scooted to the edge of the mattress. They can penetrate you with your legs up against their chest. The key is to keep your legs straight so they're not pushed back against your tummy and chest, which might not feel so great. However, you can easily modify this position by wrapping your legs around their waist or simply having them hold your thighs while your legs extend straight out behind the giver. If you lie on your stomach instead, you'll be in the Superwoman position.

Deep Impact

This sex position for larger lovers is somewhere between the legs-on-shoulder style and Missionary position. Instead of lying on top of you, your mate kneels and raises your hips so that your butt rests on their thighs. This brings your vagina/ass closer to the folic, which should make penetration easier. This position is great for deep penetration. You can leave your feet against their chest/shoulders, wrap your legs around them like in the Drill sex position or even bend at the knees and let your feet lie flat on the bed if your legs are long enough to do so.

WHAT IF THE GIVER IS BIGGER?

Get on top! When your giver is on top, their folic might be obscured. But when they lie on their back, their weight shifts in a way that gives you better access to it. You might realize that there is more access to the full length in this position. You can also do Reverse Cowgirl, where you are facing away from the giver. Unless your partner has a smaller folic that doesn't work well for Cowgirl style, you've got nothing to worry about. And that can often be fixed by placing a pillow or two beneath their hips to raise their hips up.

Even if you're much bigger than they are, you're not going to hurt them or do any lasting damage. Although, if you're too reluctant to climb on top, you might not be doing any favors to your sex life and relationship. One of the main reasons you may not want to get on top because you are afraid of how you will look. Yes, things might hang out a little more and jiggle as you move. But your partner knows what you look like, and they have already chosen to have sex with you. If they ask you to be on top, *they want you there!*

BUILDING SELF CONFIDENCE

Confidence is derived from two areas of self-evaluation. They must look at their own self-esteem and self-perception to build self-confidence. Individuals need to do self-evaluations in these areas in order to come out on the other side confidant in being a sexual being. This will make you capable of having intense orgasms and a healthy sex life at any size.

Having confidence in yourself about how you present and behave as a sexual partner is definitely going to improve your orgasm. Go inward and determine your level of self-esteem. Do you have self-esteem? Do you understand your worth? Do you know your value as a sex partner? These questions will build your confidence in realizing your image has very little to do with your value. Everyone should explore and enjoy orgasms and your body size should not hold anyone back from doing that. Build confidence in yourself so that you can rest assured that how you present is just fine.

The same goes with your perception of yourself. Are you a sexual being? Do you believe you can be a pleasant mate? What insights can you identify about yourself that will help improve your confidence? These viewpoints of yourself are going to again, build confidence in yourself. Imagine being able to do a striptease for your mate to kick off a great sex session.

All You Need to Know About Strap-Ons

A strap-on dildo (also strap-on, or dildo harness) is a dildo designed to be worn, usually with a harness, during sexual activity. Harnesses and dildos are made in a wide variety of styles, with variations in how the harness fits the wearer, how the dildo attaches to the harness, as well as various features intended to facilitate stimulation of the wearer or a sexual partner.

A strap-on dildo can be used for a wide variety of sexual activities, including vaginal sex, anal sex, oral sex, or solo or mutual masturbation. Sexual lubricant can be used to ease insertion, and strap-on dildos can be used by people of any gender or sexuality.

The principal feature of any strap-on setup is the attachment—the dildo used to penetrate the other partner. While there's a huge array of different dildos available, most are attached to the harness in one of several ways. All methods have tradeoffs, and many couples will have different harnesses depending on which type of dildo they want to use.

Many designs of strap-on have various features to increase the stimulation of the wearer. Some harnesses intentionally leave the genital area and anus open (either intentionally with an opening in the material or by the design simply not having any straps that would cover it), which allows any toy to be used for the stimulation of the wearer or even for the wearer to be penetrated while wearing the strap-on. This can often be useful when the partners wish to switch roles during their play, as the strap-on can be put on beforehand without interfering or needing to be taken off for play to continue.

HISTORY

The Kama Sutra includes mention of dildos (darshildo in Hindi) made from a wide variety of materials and used by hand, with ties (straps), or in a harness.

Female-female dildo usage in ancient China has been documented, but it is not clear if this was double-dildos, strap-on dildos, or just a simple dildo being used by one woman on another. An 1899 report by Haberlandt documented current and historical use of double-ended dildos in Zanzibar. This being one of the few historical documents of this kind. In ancient Greece, dildos were made of stone or padded leather, and some evidence shows the aforementioned leather was used to make a harness and olive oil used for anal penetration.

A 19th-century Chinese painting shows a woman using a dildo strapped to her shoe, showing that creative use of strap-ons was already well underway. A double-penetration dildo was found in ancient France, but its use is lost to time. Many artifacts from the Upper Paleolithic have been found that appear to be dildos, including a double «baton» with a hole in the middle, theorized to be for a strap to hold it to a wearer. It is likely, the history of the strap-on parallels the history of the dildo, and given the age of many discoveries, is a long history.

HARNESS MATERIALS

Harnesses are available in many different materials, and the choice of which to use depends greatly on individual preference.

Synthetic

These are harness made by chemical synthesis in order to imitate a natural product. These products are easy to clean and tend to last longer than natural products.

O-ring harness

Nylon webbing and soft foam-like synthetic leather are common, relatively affordable, and very durable. Synthetic harnesses are relatively easy to clean and require relatively little maintenance. Some, such as the Spare Parts harness, are machine washable.

Leather

Leather is comfortable and adjusts to the wearer's body, but still is strong. Leather is harder to clean and requires more work to maintain than other materials.

Cloth

Cloth is used mostly for clothing harnesses such as corsets and other lingerie, although it is occasionally used by extremely inexpensive harnesses.

Plastic

Plastic harness has little flexibility, making them the least comfortable of all the materials. They are easy to wipe clean and can be great for beginners or those into water sports.

Clear Plastic Harness

Some harnesses are made with soft plastic, such as flexible vinyl. These are often available in colors besides traditional black and maybe completely transparent (not possible with other materials). They may be less comfortable than other materials and may be difficult to make fit well; however, they are very easy to clean and fairly robust.

Latex, Rubber, PVC

Latex harnesses usually cover the entire area, rather than just using straps. They tend to be medium-priced and have a limited lifespan, especially if used with oil-based lubricants. Latex can require much care, such as special cleaners or shiners to keep it from turning dry and dusty. Latex harnesses may or may not have the dildo(s) molded as part of the harness, and in either case, they tend to be floppy due to the flexibility of the latex. Similar harnesses are also available made of rubber or PVC and are similar to latex harnesses, although PVC tends to be much less flexible and elastic.

Molded Straps

Inexpensive dildo with molded snaps. Some very cheap "strap-on dildos" have straps or attachments for straps directly molded into the material of the dildo. This design is very flimsy and is only used on the cheapest products. They are essentially useless for the traditional purpose of a strap-on dildo (one partner penetrating another using a dildo in a position similar to a penis) but can be strapped around chairs and other objects for a variety of other activities.

Pleasure for the wearer of the strap-on generally comes from pressure against the genitals, particularly the clitoris, during use and from psychological arousal.

HARNESS TYPES

The first part of a strap-on setup is the harness, which connects the dildo to the wearer's body, usually in a position similar to that of a male's genitals. A good harness should be sturdy yet comfortable and is often designed to provide stimulation for the wearer. Many types of harnesses are available, with different features and drawbacks. Some dildos do not need a harness or are built onto one; for these, please see the sections on dildo types and dildo attachment methods.

A two-strap harness

A 2-strap harness, in its most basic form, is similar to a G-string. One strap goes around the wearer's waist, like a belt, while the other goes between the wearer's legs and connects to the other strap in the middle at the lower back. While these are simple, many people find them uncomfortable because the strap rubs against the anus and other areas, and they sometimes do not hold the dildo very firmly, causing it to sag, flop, twist, or squeak.

Three-strap

Three-strap harnesses have one strap around the wearer's waist, but instead of one strap between the legs, they have two straps, one around each thigh, rejoining the first strap near the front. This design leaves the genitals and anus uncovered and attaches the dildo more firmly, giving the wearer more control. Not everyone finds this design comfortable, and sometimes they are difficult to fit properly, and tend to slip.

Corsets and other clothing items

Strap-on harnesses built into various clothing items are available, most often as a corset or other item of lingerie. Some are designed to be worn underneath normal clothing for quick use (if done with the dildo in place, either to give the appearance of a penis or to be able to quickly initiate intercourse, this is sometimes called packing), while others take advantage of the additional strength and sturdiness an item of clothing can provide over a few straps, or just to integrate the strap-on into an erotic outfit.

Body locations

Harnesses are not limited to the crotch, and indeed many types are available for other body parts. A popular one is a thigh harness, which attaches a dildo to the wearer's thigh (or other parts of the legs or arms, though this is much less common), allowing for many unique positions, as penetration is no longer limited to what could be done with a penis. Another unusual design attaches a dildo to the chin of the wearer, allowing vaginal penetration while performing anilingus or vice versa. Also, an additional design is a gag-style harness, in which a gag is inserted into the wearer's mouth, and a dildo protrudes at the other end.

Vacuum Seal

Vac-u-lock plug and powder lubricant. Used primarily by Doc Johnson, Vac-u-lock dildos have a rippled hollow in their base, which fits onto a matching plug on the harness or other toy. Powdered lubricant is used on the plug to facilitate removal. The advantage of this design is that the dildo is firmly attached and cannot easily rotate and does not tend to flop downwards or slip like ring harnesses. There is also a wide variety of other devices the dildos can be attached to, such as handles and inflatable balls. The disadvantage is the relatively low availability and high cost of compatible attachments. Several brands have non-compatible clones of the Vac-u-lock system, but dildos and accessories for them are virtually unavailable.

For Vac-u-lock harnesses, one or two additional Vac-u-lock plugs are mounted on the inside of the harness, allowing any Vac-u-lock attachment to be used. Most Vac-u-lock harnesses that have the connectors for internal plugs come with two plug-shaped Vac-u-lock attachments, a smaller one for anal use and a larger one for vaginal use. Like other types of harnesses, both plugs may be used at once and often are separately adjustable on the strap to fit the wearer's body.

Strapless

A recent design is a strapless strap-on, designed to be held in a vagina or anus with an egg-shaped bulb and thus not to require the use of a harness. This differs from a double dildo where both ends are phallic, and a harness is required. The Feeldoe is a strapless dildo which was patented by Melissa Mia Kain in 1997. Advantages of this design are that it can be used spontaneously, that it provides deep internal thrusting to both partners, and that the lack of harness makes it more comfortable. Disadvantages are that the eggs do not prevent rotation or droop, leading to a reduced amount of control unless a harness is employed anyway; a requirement for strong muscles; and the practice needed to become familiar with its use. Many strapless strap ons can also be used with a harness when partners want to increase control. Not all harnesses are suitable for strapless strap ons. It is highly recommended that you use a strap-on with a very adjustable O-ring or a two-hole harness.

O-Ring Harness with Wide-Base Dildo

The most common means of holding the dildo to the harness is to have an opening or ring in the harness through which a wide-based dildo is inserted. Inexpensive harnesses tend to just have a round hole in the fabric or leather, while more expensive ones will use a steel or rubber ring. The advantage of this method is that dildos which fit are widely available and inexpensive, and even many dildos not meant for harness use will work in one of these harnesses, such as most dildos with testicles. The major disadvantage is the dildo is often held loosely (especially on cheap harnesses) and tends to flop downwards, and the dildo often can rotate in use.

SPECIALTY FUNCTIONS

Inflatable Enema Nozzle

Many specialty dildos are available, such as ones that expand when an attached inflator bulb is squeezed, simulate ejaculation by releasing warm water on demand when a reservoir is compressed, or function as enema nozzles, allowing an enema to be given while using the strap-on for anal intercourse. Inflatable dildos generally expand in girth when inflated (they usually come with a simple hand-squeeze inflator bulb), allowing the dildo to keep expanding during intercourse as the receiver slowly stretches, giving a unique completely filled feeling which is hard to obtain using normal dildos.

Ejaculating dildos contain a squeeze bulb or other reservoir, which when filled with hot water beforehand, allows the wearer to "cum" into the receiver at the proper moment. Enema nozzle dildos contain tubing connections, and when used for anal penetration (most often with silicone lube, as water-soluble lube would quickly break down when combined with an enema), allow the receiver to receive an enema during intercourse.

Some BDSM mistresses specialize in offering this service. A relatively new product in this field is dildos with electrodes for erotic electrostimulation, further increasing the range of sensations the receiver can experience.

DILDOS

The most noticeable feature of any strap-on setup is the dildo used. A wide variety of dildos are available, and while the choices may be limited by the type of harness in use, generally one can choose from several common types. This section discusses the shape and features of the penetrating end of the dildo, not of the entire dildo or how it›s attached, which can be found in the section on dildo attachment methods for the double dildo and strapless dildo.

Standard

A standard dildo with crotchless Vac-u-lock harness. The standard dildo has a non-tapered or slightly tapered shaft and often has an enlarged head, similar to a penis. The shaft may be slightly curved, but if it is strongly curved, it is often classified as a g-spot/prostate dildo as well. This type is by far the most popular, both for vaginal and anal use, although some beginners prefer a probe-type dildo. Depending on the type of harness the dildo is meant for, it may have molded testicles as part of the base, which many people say gives more pleasure and helps keep the dildo from "bottoming out." Standard dildos are the most common by a large margin and are available in virtually any length and width, material, texture, etc.

Probe

A combination probe and g-spot dildo with a Vac-u-lock harness. A probe dildo is often highly tapered, and many resemble a cone in overall shape or may have a narrow diameter its entire length, although ones resembling an elongated butt plug are also common, their defining feature being a bulb in the middle which tapers down again towards the harness before flaring wider. These dildos are often advertised as being for beginners, especially newcomers to pegging, who may find a narrow, tapered dildo easier to start with if they have never had anal penetration before. Many people find that once they are familiar with the activity, the probe dildos are inadequate and unsatisfying, and purchase a standard dildo to use with their harness. Due to this, many kits include both a probe dildo and a standard dildo, so it is not necessary to purchase another.

G-Spot and Prostate

Dildos designed for g-spot or prostate stimulation often have a sharp upwards curve at the head or gradual but still strong curvature the entire length. When used in many sexual positions, the curve causes strong pressure against the g-spot in women or the prostate in men. Some men report that strong prostate stimulation is important for an anal orgasm, while others report it as a distraction rather than a help. When using one of these dildos for the first time, care should be taken at first to make sure it's comfortable for the receiver, as the strong bend can be difficult to insert or control. For many positions, such as doggy style, the curved tip should point downwards, as otherwise it points in the wrong direction for either g-spot or prostate stimulation.

Penis Extensions

Hollow dildos are often sold as penis extensions, but the most common use is for men with erectile dysfunction. The penis is inserted into the hollow inside of the dildo; then the harness is put on, allowing the man to penetrate his partner with the dildo, the thrusting of which is transferred to his penis.

Upon Objects

Inflatable ball with Vac-u-lock plug and attached dildo. Harnesses are available to attach dildos to just about any household object, allowing for many creative uses. A dildo could be attached to a chair, bed, or any other item of furniture and penetrate someone during other activities, with or without a partner. Another item, while not technically a harness, but worth mentioning, is an inflatable ball, usually 9 to 18 inches (250 to 500 mm) diameter, made of sturdy rubber designed to support the weight of one or two people, with an attachment for a dildo on it. This allows many unique positions, such as double penetration for a woman by lying face down on the ball for vaginal penetration while her partner penetrates her anally doggy style, which is much more effective than a solid object due to the "bounce" of the ball. These inflatable balls are also quite popular for solo use.

Vibrating and Rotating

Multi-function dildo with rotating beads and vibrating egg. Some dildos, especially recent ones, may have rotating beads along the shaft, a wiggling shaft, vibrating ticklers or other clitoral stimulation devices, or other features to give more pleasure to the user. While their effectiveness is a matter of opinion, they are becoming increasingly popular. An inexpensive design is basically a standard rabbit vibrator designed for harness use (often exactly the same toy with a slightly different base), while more expensive dildos are designed from the ground-up for harness use and are usually superior. Rotating beads provide extra stimulation of the vulva and vaginal opening when used for vaginal penetration or stimulation of the anus when used for anal penetration, while the various clitoral stimulation devices are generally intended only for vaginal intercourse. These dildos are often bulky or heavy, and like all other vibrators, need a power source (usually batteries in a pack that clips onto the harness or slips into a pocket on it), but can provide additional stimulation for those who desire it.

Double penetration

Double penetration dildos are generally two dildos molded onto a common base, designed for simultaneous vaginal and anal penetration or simultaneous vagina and vagina penetration, not to be confused with a man using a strap-on along with his penis for double penetration. A typical double-penetration dildo has a longer, thicker main shaft for vaginal penetration and a shorter, thinner, often more curved shaft for anal penetration. Although rare, dildos with the anal shaft being equally as large as the vaginal shaft are available for women who find a larger anal dildo more satisfying. These dildos tend to greatly limit the possible positions they are used in, as the angle must be right for both vaginal and anal penetration when thrusting; however, they can provide a unique experience for couples to try.

EXTERNAL STIMULATION

Jelly-coated vibrating egg

Some harnesses and dildos provide raised bumps or other features designed to rub against the clitoris of a female wearer, either attached to the inside of the harness or on the back of the base of the dildo. Harnesses that work with such dildos must have an open back, where the base of the dildo presses directly against the woman's body. As high-quality harnesses usually have padding or other means of attaching the dildo to the harness than a simple opening. These features are usually only seen on low-quality, inexpensive dildos. They provide only limited stimulation, and while better than nothing, are usually considered inferior to other types.

Vibrators

Another means of providing stimulation to the wearer is a vibrating egg, "clit blaster", vibrating gel pads or whiskers, or other device mounted on the inside of the strap on. These are almost always intended for use by women, as the external vibrator is rarely positioned well nor provides stimulation to males. These devices provide external stimulation to the clitoris, vulva, and other parts of the vaginal opening, but do not provide any penetrative stimulation or anal stimulation.

INTERNAL STIMULATION

Double-ended attachments

While a double dildo obviously would provide stimulation to the wearer as well, the standard straight dildo is very poorly suited for harness use. To overcome this, many dildos are available for harness use that have an offset in the middle, with the main attachment and a smaller vaginal attachment for the wearer having a flat vertical section between them. This way, the main attachment is at a good angle and position for thrusting, while its movement is transmitted directly to the vaginal plug and clitoris of the wearer.

Strap-on harness with dual internal plugs

Many of the "professional" harnesses have one or two plugs (vaginal, anal, or both) on the inside of the harness to penetrate the wearer. Harnesses made for men usually only come with the anal plug, while ones for women come with both plugs, which most women report provides the most pleasure using one.
While a plug can be used in combination with most any harness, just by inserting the plugs before putting on the harness, all the harness tends to do is push the plugs in, and not move them as to provide stimulation when the wearer thrusts.

A common type consists of an opening or rubber ring with a cloth or leather back, similar to what might be used to hold the main dildo to the front of the harness, but positioned over the anus, vagina, or ones for both. A dildo/plug with a wide base is inserted through the ring, then when the harness is put on, the material pulls tight against it, holding it firm

Double-ended/sided hands and strap free dildos

The latest technological achievement is totally new kind of strapless strap-on. Due to the shape of the dildo, thrusting on the main dildo translates to lateral movement of the plug, providing great stimulation to the wearer.

The shape of the plug allows it to be used without a harness in many instances. It can also allow a penis owner to perform a double penetration while being anal plugged himself, all with only a single toy.

What to Do with the Rest of Him

So, you have performed oral, rode them crazy and handled the penis like a stick shift. What else is there to do...to do... to do? Much! Add some fresh and new moves that can spruce up what you have tried and tested before. The body has so many erotic points to be explored.

These zones are referred to as the erogenous zones and are places or areas on the body that cause arousal and extend, expands, and enlighten additional methods to orgasm. From the sides and back of the neck, armpits, chest, inner arms and thighs, a tickle, a stroke, or a lick uses the sensory of anticipation to create a sexual response. Everyone may not enjoy this, often for them, it may tickle, hurt, or simple turn them off. Often a mutual attraction must exist.

There are different responses to areas that have hair then non-hair zones. The hair on the body grows due to testosterone and the surface is known as the epithelium. There are several different representations of these surfaces. Where there is less hair, it is reported to have more sensitivity. This is because the epithelium is bare. (i.e., inner arm)

You can blindfold or use lube for any action you do on the body. Be mindful that anticipation is the goal of adding a sense of arousal. Be prepared for any reaction and follow the lead of the person as you go ahead and experiment.

IMAGINATION

This isn't a tangible thing you can touch; you can still stimulate this part of them. Let them have some time to consider your touch before your fingers arrive on their skin. The ultimate tease. Whisper in their ear softly and tell them all the things you are going to do to them without touching a hair on their body. Just pretend like you're sexting and say those things to them in real life.

ABDOMEN AND NAVEL

Many people find stimulation (kissing, biting, scratching, tickling, caressing) of the abdomen to be pleasurable, especially close to the pubic region. It can cause strong arousal in individuals, in some even stronger than stimulation of the genitals. The navel is one of the many erogenous zones that has heightened sensitivity. The navel and the region below when touched by the finger or the tip of the tongue results in the production of erotic sensations.

SPINE

Known as the sacrum, the base of the spine is an erotic spot to lick, suck and massage for arousal.

FINGERS

The tips of their fingers have many nerves and respond to even the lightest of touches. Human fingertips are the second-most sensitive parts of the body, after the tongue. Placing your finger or fingers into their mouth and massage the inner jaws, tongue, roof without reaching too far back to cause them to gag. Allow them to suck on your fingers and moan as they do it to increase stimulation with touch, sound, and visual enticement. Brush your tongue along the fingertips. Pull their fingers into your mouth much as you would a penis. Use saliva to create a wetness while rolling your tongue over and around the fingers.

ARMPITS

The erogenous zone of the armpits is a very individualize sensitivity experience. Because its normal-haired dense texture, the nerve sensitivity is different for everyone. However, you use intense and suspenseful touches and strokes; you should elicit some arousal. Don't go too light as to tickle them. If using your mouth, you should be prepared to apply pressure based on the amount of hair that is there. Be sure your mate is clean unless your fetish is the musk of the area. Apply lots of pressure first and soften the touch based on their response.

ARMS

The softer skin of the inner arm and the crease that is the mid-arm bend are very sensitive to hand, feet, or mouth manipulation. Vigorous kneading and light kiss can induce erection and/or ejaculation without touching the penis. Where the arm bends is sensitive due to the lack of hair in the area. Obese people may have less sensitivity and folks with thinner skin may find the touches painful or uncomfortable at least.

HAIR

There are nerve endings on their scalp that are attached to the rest of their body, and when their hair is gently pulled when they are kissed or held, it sends stimulation to the rest of their body. While kissing, try running the tips of your fingers through the hair, over their scalp gently, then a bit harder with a tug. If they react with small sounds and pleasure moans, pull harder, then let go before they want you to. This playful tease with drive them legit crazy.

THE FEET IN GENERAL

Because of the concentration of nerve endings in the sole and digits of the human foot, and possibly due to the proximity between the area of the brain dealing with tactile sensations from the feet and the area dealing with sensations from the genitals, the sensations produced by both the licking of the feet and sucking of toes can be pleasurable to some people. Similarly, massaging the sole of the foot can produce similar stimulation. Many people are extremely ticklish in the foot area, especially on the soles. There's a reason why reflexology massages are so popular. Be gentle, and with adding pressure can be erotic for some. You can apply pressure from your tongue or fingertips to give a massage that advances with their response. Start by using some massage oil and massaging the feet, especially the arch of the foot.

TOES

Shrimpin' anyone? Yes, this is what it's called when you suck on your partner's toes. This is so erotic because feet are a nonconventional hotbed of sensation just waiting for some stimulation. During sexy foreplay, move your kisses teasingly down their body until you're all the way down to their feet. Suck on your partner's toes—or even lick the bottom of their foot arch.

BUTT CHEEK

They are going to be extra sensitive here. Striking their butt cheek, even lightly, tends to stimulate the whole area. Think of it like a slow vibration flowing through their insides. If your mate is open to a little spank play, this is great to do while they are on top of you in any variation of missionary. Squeeze their booty when they are hitting just the right spot; give them a quick spank if you're both into it. A great act to try is surfing, a baby oil butt ride. Simple and erotic. Oil or other wet substances in the sex act is a fetish. Most call it sloshing. Place towels or additional sheets on the bed/surface and generously pour baby oil on your entire front and their entire body. Use your body to massage theirs, rub, apply pressure, stroke, and knead their body to orgasm. Be aware of the oil ingredients BEFORE using your mouth.

THE PHILTRUM

The small groove above the lips has long been considered an erogenous zone. Philtrum, translates from the Latin word for "love potion." To stimulate the philtrum, plant a very soft kiss on this area right before running your tongue down the groove to meet their upper lip.

INNER THIGH

Since the inner thigh is so close to the genitals, even without the sensation of touch, just being in that area is sure to get them anticipating what's next. Take your time to kiss and lick their inner thigh before going to touch the genitals when performing oral. Tease them and experiment with your lips. You can go from light fluttering kisses to harder sucking. It may tickle or it may feel like butterflies in the belly. Use long strokes from knee to groin. DO NOT touch the genitals, including the anus. Be sure to stay focus on the inner skin with a soft tongue and the rest of the legs with a little more pressure.

BOTTOM LIPS

The lips in general, are one of the most sensitive parts of the body. Take your time while kissing. There's a reason why nibbling and variation in pressure can drive you over the edge when done correctly. Gentle and with added pressure can be erotic for some. You can apply pressure from your tongue or fingertips to give a massage that advances with their response. Nibbling their bottom lips and possibly even going for a harder bite. The sensations of going from a tender kiss to some teeth will surprise your mate and excite the brain.

THE OUTSIDE OF THEIR LOWER LIP

The area between the lower lip and the chin is an erogenous zone for most. It is packed with extra sensitive nerve receptors. Suck their lower lip into your mouth the next time you're making out and use the tip of your tongue to stroke this under-lip area. That motion stimulates the whole erogenous zone in a teasing way, which will put them on the erotic edge. Keeping the lower lip inside yours magnifies the sensation. It'll feel as if electric currents are shooting from your lips straight to their genitals.

V-LINES

The V-zone is a hot bed of pleasure for your partner; not only is it a turn-on that they have front-row tickets to watch you stimulate them, but it's an easy pit stop to make on the way to downtown. Have them lay on their back while you straddle them and give them what they really want. Starting from their belly button, use your fingers and nails to trace a line down from the happy trail, stopping before you hit total groin. Then retrace your steps but use your tongue to trace a V shape from their hips to the right above the genitals. Draw it out and really tease them until they can't take it any longer.

NECK

The Adam's apple is an erogenous zone; thought behind this stems from how the thyroid (just below the Adam's apple) is closely linked to the sex organs. The clavicle area and the back of the neck have sensitive nerve endings that can be stroked or licked to arousal. Suck, (hickey?) kiss and squeeze the neck. Have them lie on their back and literally just suck the Adam's apple. Keep your tongue flat and light, not too much pressure! For all individuals you can massage the area with wide circular motions to ensure you're hitting that T-spot of the thyroid.

NIPPLES

Nipples are even more sensitive than other body parts since for some; they may not be used to having them touched so often. Touch them, however, and you'll send shock waves of pleasure radiating throughout the body. The areola and nipple have concentrated nerve tissue and its ducts swell with arousal, causing the nipple to get hard. Concentrated attention to the nipple may result in an increase of oxytocin and prolactin that causes a significant amount of arousal, specifically in the genitals. Use your breasts/chest and nipples as well as your hands and fingers to stimulate nipple arousal. Have them lie on their back and slowly lick from the areola inward, like an ice-cream cone but never touching tongue to nipple yet. Get closer and closer until you flick the nipple with your tongue and then gently bite it. If you want to be extra, you can suck on an ice cube beforehand for more sensation.

THE DIP UNDER THEIR ANKLE

This is the spot that may get bruised when you wear new shoes. There is a fingertip sized pressure point that holds enormous passion potential. This spot is linked to the sex organs and pressing it releases energy, producing feelings of pleasure. While in reverse-cowgirl, grab their feet and pulse each pressure point in rhythm with your thrusts. Try this right before they are about to climax to really blow their mind.

LOWER BACK

The pudendal nerve that stimulates all the groin areas is located here, at the bottom of the spinal cord. Have your partner take their shirt off and lay on their stomach with their arms by their side. Keep their pants on but pull them down a few inches for a tantalizing never-nude experience. Lightly run your fingers or anxiety-ravaged cuticles down across the lower back, stopping before you hit ass cheek. Do this until you can't stand but undress and finish with orgasm.

EARLOBES

You may know the feeling you get from someone whispering in your ear. Playing with the earlobes can be very sensual and send shivers down the spine. Kiss your partner across their shoulder, up the neck, and stopping right before you hit the ear. Do this to both sides. When they are right about to lose it, start kissing the earlobe, and use your tongue to bring the earlobe into your mouth. Play around with gentle nibbles, tongue, etc. Be careful not to touch any other part of their body while doing this and see how wild they get from you just touching the earlobes. A great place to caress, kiss, lick, bite, or suck.

THE RAPHE

The raphe is the dividing line that runs across the middle of their genitalia from the anus to the tip of the penis, down over the perineum, scrotum, and shaft. Use your tongue to trace over the line and teasing them into your mouth. Try using a lubed-up bullet vibrator like the We-Vibe Tango to trace along the line as well, while you breathe, lick, and suck in conjunction with the vibrator.

PERINEUM

The perineum is REALLY sensitive and worth exploring. This patch of skin is located between the balls and the anus and between the vagina and anus. Before they enter you in missionary, reach between their legs and touch the genitals. Then press your knuckles gently into this spot and start massaging. Right as they are about to orgasm, push your knuckles a little deeper to extend the fireworks.

SHAFT

While you may have mastered the typical handy and blow job, try to spice things up with something totally uncharted like a reverse finger job. Make two tight rings around the penis with your thumb and index finger (like you're doing the okay hand symbol 👌), stacking them one on top of the other in the middle of the shaft. Twist the rings in opposite directions moving from the middle to the top and base of the shaft at the same time. Remember to use lube.

THE HEAD OF THE PENIS

As the most sensitive part of the penis, the head can be a fickle art to master. It can be tricky to get the right level of pressure, so you send them soaring into ecstasy but without recoiling in sensory overload. Give them a lipstick blow job—aka where you brush your closed but relaxed lips against the head of the penis like you're applying lipstick. Hold the shaft with your fingers, but not in a fist (avoid holding the penis like a microphone). Vary the sensations by opening your mouth a bit and rubbing the head between them.

THE SEAM OF THE TESTICLES

Testicles have a seam that keeps the scrotums in separate sacks. It is a nerve rich pleasure trail that runs top to bottom along the scrotum. Cradle the balls in one hand while gently pressing the first two fingertips of your other hand into the top of the crease (close to where the testicles connect to the base of the penis). Then trace downward with your fingers until you reach the bottom of the scrotum. Don't forget to be gentle!

FRENULUM

The F-spot is the little nubbin of flesh underneath the crown of the penis connecting the head to the shaft. It's often overlooked because it's part of the undercarriage; there's a bundle of nerves at this point that, when touched, can set off an amazing chain reaction of rapture. The next time you're going down, hold the penis steady with one hand while really giving the crown your all. Each time you circle your tongue around to the frenulum, flick it a few times with your tongue stiffened, and then relax and go back to licking the crown.

I hope you try and implement some of this into your lovemaking sessions. Often sex seems redundant when you only do the same two things to the penis owner. Learn to make love to the entire body. The heightened arousal will help them to achieve better, more intense orgasms.

Anal Orgasm

Anal orgasms are common very pleasurable orgasms. They are popular among men due to the prostate. Stimulating the prostate by gently inserting a finger straight forward and massage the glands will bring about an anal orgasm. For women, simply rubbing the outside of the anal opening and placing a finger inside can cause an orgasm. The key is to use lube. The anus DOES NOT self-lubricate; therefore, lube is mandatory. The tissue is extremely sensitive and easy to tear which could lead to infection.

Who says anal orgasms are only for people with penises? You can still get off through anal play by indirectly stimulating the G-spot through the wall shared between the rectum and vagina. But remember: You must, must, *must* use lube, as your anus doesn't self-lubricate naturally.

Start massaging the outside and inside of your anal opening, then slowly and gently insert your finger or sex toy into your anus. Switch between a circular and in-and-out motion as you penetrate your anus. Go faster as the pleasure begins to build until you're ready to finish. Experiment with toys! Vibrators, plugs, anal beads, and massagers can intensify your orgasm tenfold.

Anal play can be enjoyed by anyone of any gender or orientation. Anal play can include placing fingers or tongue inside/around the anus. This is called rimming. Placing a penis, dildo, or sex toy inside the anus. Putting a hand inside of the anus (fisting). You should be sure to use lots of lube to ease the entry process.

It is normal to practice this act. Because of the number of nerve endings in the rectum, it is very pleasurable. Analingus or rimming is the licking or oral-anal contact, touching with fingers or other body parts or objects. You should keep your mind open to giving or receiving this sort of play.

WHAT YOU SHOULD KNOW

- You can perform anal sex on yourself. Some prefer to do this so that they know what to expect and what pleases them in anal play.

- Communication is key when anal play is on the table. Be sure to talk to your partner throughout the act. Make sure you and your partner are both comfortable with everything you want to do.

- Do not attempt entry without a good water-based lube. Lube is your best friend so use it liberally. Be gentle; the tissues that make up the anus are very sensitive and tear easily.

- You and your partner are in control of your own comfort level. Be sure to check in with each other often to be sure everyone is still having fun.

- Anal play will not cause you to have constipation, hemorrhoids, or diarrhea. If you do have these conditions, you should wait until they clean up before playing.

- Be sure to wash your hands and use a new condom when switching from anal play to your other genitals. Use a dental dam or condoms when sharing toys or rimming.

- Be sure to use good, high-quality toys. ALWAYS use a condom. You may want to start small and work your way up to your pleasure point. Covering cheap anal toys with condoms, contrary to popular belief, doesn't stop nasty chemicals from seeping into your skin.

- You can definitely catch an STI even if there is no penetration. Know your health status and be comfortable enough to discuss this with your partner.

- There can be odd sounds and/or poop which is normal. You may want to shower before or during to keep things clean and appealing. It does not have to be messy. You can put down a towel or plastic sheet or have wipes handy before you play.

- Relax and take your time. This is not an act that should be done quickly. Be aware of what feels good and stop anything if it does not feel right mentally or physically. Breathe, relax. If pain does occur, stop, and evaluate what is going on at the moment.

ANAL PLAY AND THE LAW

Be sure to know about any laws in your neck of the woods regarding anal play. In many countries, the act is criminalized although many of these laws have been overturned and not enforced. In 1986 The US Supreme Court ruled that the US Constitution bars a state from banning anal play. Currently, only 10 states have laws prohibiting sodomy, penalizing up to fifteen years in prison. Only four states have laws that address same-sex anal play.

In 2003, the US Supreme Court put down the Texas same-sex sodomy law. Citing that the private sexual conduct is protected. Knowing the status of your state is helpful, but again, what you do in the privacy of your own home is no longer anybody's business.

Surveys suggest that more people are exploring anal play in some way. Interest in anal eroticism does not always include penetration and doesn't have to. It may not be a part of a healthy fun sex life.

THE ANUS

The opening of the anus holds the highest concentration of nerve endings. The anal opening known as the sphincter muscles, anal canal and prostate gland make up the rectum. The feelings of fullness or pressure is the pleasure or arousal aspect. Placing pressure on the ventral wall of the anus, just a couple inches in will stimulate the prostate gland. The tip of the internal clitoral body can be stimulated through the anus as well.

PLAY SAFELY

As stated, the lining of the anus is very sensitive and easy to damage. Be sure to play safe by taking things slow, listening to your body and the reactions of your partner. Anything that you place near the anus should be smooth; this includes your fingernails. It is best to keep them short and rounded. Use toys that are unbreakable, flexible, smooth, clean, and comfortable in size. Use a toy with a flared base. Anything that can slip from your grasp may not be retrievable. You may have heard of stories in which folks have gone into emergency rooms to have items/rodents removed from their rectum/intestines.

The anus does not make its own lubrication, so be sure to use lubrication. Use a liberal amount of water-based lube each and every time you plan penetration. Lubrication can help lower the risk of tears or damage.

Be sure to keep clean. Do not move anything from the anus to the vagina. Bacteria that live safely in the anus can cause havoc in the vagina. Use fresh condoms and gloves as well as wash your hands to avoid cross-contamination. A dental dam can be an excellent blocker during oral-anal contact.

LUBES

Lube is a MUST-HAVE when playing anally. Again, the anus does not self-lubricate, and safe play always, always, always requires lube.

Lube that works quite well is water-based. It's free of stinging chemicals like glycerin and parabens and is compatible with all types of materials.

For firm toys, you may want to use a silicone lube. Although it is NOT compatible with silicone toys, the lube is a great choice for anal sex with a partner, glass, metal, or wood toys. Silicone lube is extra slick and does not dry out as quickly as water-based lubes.

ANAL TOYS

Using a toy that is completely body-safe, certified seamless silicone that may vibrate, swirl, is beaded or weighted that can take anal play to a new level.

Obviously, the goal of anal play is to experience the maximum orgasmic pleasure you can handle. Choosing toys to play with is not a simple task. There are a lot of products on the market, finding the right one for you may take some time. Here are some tips and suggestions.

There are two different types of anal toys. Prostate specific and inflatable. Prostate specific orgasms are known as the P-spot with an orgasm similar to the G-spot in females. If you were born with a penis, then you have a P-spot or prostate inside of your rectum. It is about 3 inches into the anal canal. On the front wall towards the penis and is the size of a walnut.

To use a prostate specific anal toy, you should angle the penis or toy up toward the P-spot. Once you comfortably are inside, gently angle it up as if you're reaching toward your penis through the pelvis. The receiver will feel extra full inside. They may have the urge to pee or orgasm. You may also enjoy masturbating or partnered stroking. Using a toy that vibrates intensifies the sensations. Male born givers feel the tightness of the rectum walls and can thrust their way to orgasm.

Inflatable anal toys are a great choice for some. They operate like a balloon; you insert them while they are small and then pump it up with air to stretch the sphincters and muscle of the anal canal. Always start out by pumping slowly. You do not want to force the anus open or use hard pumps to fill the toy too rapidly. Release the air by using the little valve until it's back to its original size and slide it out gently.

Flared base toys are a MUST. Anything that you place up into your rectum should have a flared base that can always be held. Many items can be sucked inside of your anus. Your muscles will suck things up into your intestines which could be life-threatening. Know that anytime you place something in, it must have a T-shaped base to hold it on the outside.

ANAL BEADS

Vagina owners can place anal beads in as their vagina is being penetrated, and penis owners can play with the beads while receiving oral or a hand job.

Anal beads have many different versions and has a ring or T shaped handle on the end of the nylon string to maintain a grasp and not lose the toy in the sphincter. They are small to medium sized and are super easy to use. They are a series of ABS plastic or silicone beads that are linked together and are used to stimulate the walls and canal of the anus. The beads start small at the insertion point and become larger at the end of the string.

Vibrating anal beads give you added sensations. Some or all of the beads can vibrate for extra sensations during anal play. You should cover the beads in a water-based lube to make insertion smoother and pleasurable.

BUTT PLUGS

Butt plugs are weighted vibrating or non-vibrating cone-shaped toys. They are usually end with a T base. As expected, the tip is smaller than the end and this makes it easier to insert.

If vibrations are too intense, you can always use the plug without turning it on until you get used to the sensation. Vibrating Butt Plugs help relax the sphincter muscles and stimulate the G-spot and P-spot. The vibrations work away muscle tightness and provide extra pleasure to the nerves in and around the anus.

Weighted butt plugs don't vibrate and are great to wear any time for pleasure anywhere. They use small sets of internal weights to create a feeling of fullness and movement while engaged. Often shaped like a torpedo, must are very comfortable to wear while engaging in other sexual positions and activities.

ANAL TOY MATERIALS

You want to choose the right material for you. There are many options on the market, and you must find those that fit your needs. Some points to keep in mind are knowing the soft materials such as PVC, latex, rubber, jelly, or silicone. Firmer materials such as ABS Plastic, glass, metals, or wood, to name a few.

The only safe soft anal toys are silicone. They are bendable, usually medical-grade first-generation silicone. Silicon is hypoallergenic and makes the toys enjoyable for all. Free from plastic softening, phthalates that are in PVC and types of rubber.

Soft materials work great for all play. Most are super flexible and move with your body. Others are stiff in the core and covered with a soft material. These materials are NOT safe for your body because the chemical compounds used to make them are unstable and can leak toxic substances, causing painful chemical burns when used internally.

Firmer materials are used for more direct, pinpointed stimulation of the P and G spots. Use a non-porous material which can be polished and coated wood, or stainless steel or alumni are great alternatives to silicone.

WHAT TO AVOID

Cheap toys are porous toys, which means that bacteria inside your rectum will begin to grow in the toy's pores. Even cleaning with antibacterial soap or cleaner can't go deep enough to fully sterilize the toy for future use.

Phthalates should be avoided altogether. They are often in soft or cheap anal toys and can adversely affect the reproductive system. These toys tend to smell like plastic and it's important to read the packaging and pay attention to the safety icons before using the toy.

CLEAN YOUR BUTT AND YOUR TOYS

Toy Cleaners are specifically made to kill bacteria and clean your toy for another use. You can use warm water and antibacterial soap, but these cleaners are made with the toy in mind. Spray some on the toy and wipe it down with a warm cloth and dry with a clean towel. Toys should be stored in cool, dry places.

Boiling toys depends on the manufacture's guidelines. Heat-resistant anal toys can be sterilized through boiling. Submerge your toy in a pot of boiling water for 3 minutes. Vibrating toys should not be boiled.

ENEMAS AND DOUCHES

It's highly unlikely that you'll encounter any poop during play if you've got a normally functioning digestive system, as fecal matter doesn't usually hang around in the lower part of your rectum. Rinsing with water is a surefire way for you to feel 100% certain that you're clean and ready for play.

Enemas and douches work in the same way basically. You fill them with lukewarm water, gently squirt the water into your rectum and then sit on a toilet and let nature runs its course.

A douche holds around a cup's worth of water, so this option is easier for a quick rinse of the area immediately inside your anus. An enema bag holds anywhere from 1 cup to around a half gallon. The more water you flush into your body, the more fecal matter will be loosened, so take your time and let your intestines work

Regardless of which option you choose, always practice on a day when you don't plan on having anal sex at all. It often takes a few hours for your body to fully flush itself from an anal water cleanse. Once you get the hang of it, use a small amount of water in a douche about 45 minutes to 1 hour before you have sex if you're feeling the need to get extra fresh.

SHARING YOUR ANAL TOYS

Should you? Can you? Like most sex toys, sharing them increases your risk of giving or receiving any STI/Ds. Always play safe, and it's best if you do not share your anal toys. As well, bacteria like E. coli and parasites can easily be transmitted through shared toys. If you happen to share, be sure to use a new condom each time and use a toy made from silicone.

TOY FEATURES

Body safe anal toys are hypoallergenic, non-porous and phthalates free and have several benefits. They are more hygienic because they are easier to clean and kill growing bacteria. Silicone is one of the safest forms of rubber that can be inserted. While it is porous, its pores are so small it cannot harbor bacteria.

Skin-like texture of silicone allows the toy to offer a true life-like experience. Meaning that you will feel as if the "real" thing is in there. The material warms quickly to body temperature and retains the heat, making it even more pleasurable.

Another excellent quality of silicone is its superb ability to transmit vibration. Silicone sex toys are made to transmit powerful vibration and pulsation to the clitoris, G-Spot or the prostate.

Silicone toys last longer! They come in a wide range of colors, shapes, firmness, etc., to ensure you are on top of your best anal play experiences.

Anal sex can be a lot of fun and very pleasurable. If you start out slow and work your way through the process, you will create a better experience. When you learn how your mate likes to be penetrated, you can deliver exactly what is asked for. Extra note: Once you enter and are in at the point of comfort, try not to come back out. Reentry causes the person to tense again, making the penetration painful. Take your time until you learn the process.

Your Health and Sex

Intercourse pain or dyspareunia is common for all genders. This could be for many reasons, an illness or infection or a psychological or physical problem. Sex may be uncomfortable because you are not relaxed or aroused enough. As well, some infections such as thrush and cystitis can cause painful sex.

In penis owners, painful intercourse can be caused by physical things such as: a prostate, urethra or testes infection caused by genital herpes and chlamydia. An allergic reaction to spermicide in the condom. Bending the penis during an erection can cause fibrous plaques on the upper side of the penis. This is called Peyronie's disease. Arthritis of the lower back can also cause sex to be painful.

Painful sex in vulva owners can be as simple as not having enough lubrication to having an STI. Often a lack of foreplay, a drop in estrogen after menopause, childbirth, or during breast-feeding will cause painful sex. Medications are known to affect sexual desire or arousal which can lower the amount of lubrication the vagina produces.

The following can all result in painful sex. Some are treatable and some are manageable. Some treatments for female sexual pain do require a doctor's care. If vaginal dryness is due to menopause, ask your primary doctor about estrogen creams or other prescription medications. Other causes of painful intercourse may also require prescription drugs.

- Endometriosis. This is a condition in which the tissue similar to that which lines the uterus grows outside the uterus.
- Vaginismus. This is a common condition. It involves an involuntary spasm in the vaginal muscles, sometimes caused by fear of being hurt.
- Ectopic pregnancy. This is a pregnancy in which a fertilized egg develops outside the uterus.
- Vaginal infections. These conditions are common and include yeast infections.
- Problems with the cervix (opening to the uterus). In this case, the penis can reach the cervix at maximum penetration. So, problems with the cervix (such as infections) can cause pain during deep penetration.
- Intercourse too soon after surgery or childbirth.
- Injury to the vulva or vagina. These injuries may include a tear from childbirth or from a cut (episiotomy) made in the skin area between the vagina and anus during labor.
- Problems with the uterus. These problems may include fibroids that can cause deep intercourse pain.
- Problems with the ovaries. Problems might include cysts on the ovaries.
- Pelvic inflammatory disease (PID). With PID, the tissues deep inside become badly inflamed and the pressure of intercourse causes deep pain.

- Menopause. With menopause, the vaginal lining can lose its normal moisture and become dry.

- Sexually transmitted infections. These may include genital warts, herpes sores, or other STIs.

- Vulvodynia. This refers to chronic pain that affects external sexual organs -- collectively called the vulva -- including the labia, clitoris, and vaginal opening. It may occur in just one spot or affect different areas from one time to the next. Doctors don't know what causes it, and there is no known cure. But self-care combined with medical treatments can help bring relief.

For cases of sexual pain in which there is no underlying medical cause, sexual therapy might be helpful. Some individuals may need to resolve issues such as guilt, inner conflicts regarding sex, or feelings regarding past abuse. Call a doctor if there are symptoms such as bleeding, genital lesions, irregular periods, vaginal discharge, or involuntary vaginal muscle contractions. Set up an appointment with me if there are other painful sex issues that need to be addressed.

PC MUSCLE

Knowing the power of the pubococcygeus muscles (PC muscle) will open a whole new world of sexual pleasure. Mastering this muscle can be done through performing Kegels as often as you can. A Kegel is when you tighten your butt cheeks as if you are holding in a fart and draw in your vagina as if you are stopping the urine flow. Hold for 10 counts and then release repeat. Do these at least three times a day. You really can do them anywhere as no one will know when you are doing them. All genders can perform this exercise and build up this muscle.

The PC muscle is the muscle that tells the body to release urine or seminal fluid in penis owners and because there is a lack of education when it comes to female ejaculation, it has no other name except "Female ejaculate." So, there's that.

This muscle is why you do not have to worry about peeing on someone during intercourse. The feeling is coming from aroused areas around the bladder and the fluid in the urethra tube. For vulva owners, Kegels also keep the vagina healthy. They can help penis owners have multiple orgasms.

When you do the Kegel, be sure you don't hold your breath. Breath in and out as you tense and release. Your body will automatically tense and you will find that you are holding your breath. Try your best to fight the urge and take relaxing breaths.

The Problem Could Be Medical

I can help some clients through difficulties with orgasm with various exercises. However, the issue may lie in the medical arena. Whether mentally with past traumas or barriers or via the medicine a person is on. Some of the medical side effects of medication cause problem with the sexual process.

Weston, (Weston 2018) suggests using an FDA approved device called Eros to stimulate the tissue within the vagina, which helps to increase blood flow to the genitals. This is found in sex novelty shops or online at several novelty store sites. There are also over the counter creams that may increase sensitivity and help a vulva owner reach orgasm. These are not FDA-approved yet, and you should consult a doctor before you start using it.

The benefits of the Eros Clitoral Therapy Device are the most advanced in research. It is a hand-held wand with a small, comfortable suction cup on the end. The clitoris and external genitals are stimulated. The suction increases blood flow to the genitals results in increased vaginal lubrication and enhanced ability to achieve orgasm. Eventually leading to the cure of this sexual dysfunction for a high number of clients.

Benefits of Eros Therapy Clitoral Device include:

- Greater clitoral and genital engorgement
- Increased vaginal lubrication
- Enhanced ability to achieve orgasm
- Improved overall sexual satisfaction

Female Sexual Dysfunction (FSD)

Female Sexual Dysfunction (FSD)is prevalent in 43% of American women. Due to the work done on erectile dysfunction, the call was made to address female sexual dysfunction. Sexual dysfunction is defined as "the persistent impairment of normal or usual patterns of sexual interest and/or responses". (Healio Health, 2019). FSD is characterized by "reduced or no clitoral sensation, reduced or no lubrication and difficulty or inability to experience an orgasm. It includes disorders related to arousal, orgasm, and pain, resulting in personal distress", (Healio Health. 2019). FSD was adopted by the Sexual Function Health Council of the American Foundation for Urologic Disease to include both psychogenic and organic causes of desire, arousal, orgasm, and sexual pain disorders. The following definitions were developed.

VARIOUS DEFINITIONS OF FEMALE SEXUAL DYSFUNCTION

Hypoactive sexual desire disorder

The persistent or recurrent deficiency (or absence) of sexual fantasies, thoughts and/or desire for, or receptivity to, sexual activity, which causes personal distress.

Sexual aversion disorder

The persistent or recurrent phobic aversion to and avoidance of sexual contact with a sexual partner, which causes personal distress.

Sexual Arousal Disorder

The persistent or recurrent ability to attain or maintain sufficient sexual excitement, causing personal distress. It may be expressed as a lack of subjective excitement or a lack of genital (lubrication/swelling) or other somatic responses.

Orgasmic Disorder

The persistent or recurrent difficulty, delay in, or absence of attaining orgasm following sufficient sexual stimulation and arousal, which causes personal distress.

Sexual Pain Disorders

Dyspareunia — Recurrent or persistent genital pain associated with sexual intercourse.

Vaginismus — Recurrent or persistent involuntary spasm of the musculature of the outer third of the vagina that interferes with vaginal penetration.

Non-Coital Sexual Pain Disorder — Recurrent persistent genital pain induced by non-coital sexual stimulation. Despite the common occurrence of FSD, many women may be too embarrassed or reluctant to discuss their sexual problems with their physician. In addition, physicians have had few effective treatments for FSD to prescribe. The Eros Therapy gives the physician the opportunity to prescribe a treatment for patients who complain of diminished vaginal lubrication, diminished clitoral sensation, reduced ability to achieve orgasm and lowered sexual satisfaction.

Choose now to become the best sexual version of yourself. The first step is to recognize that you are a sexual being. Regardless of your orientation, gender, or pleasure taste, you can begin to live a much more satisfying life by learning how to embrace your sexual health and learn how to navigate the conversation around your orgasm.

Sex Positions

As long as you are willing and able to keep your sex life alive and active, you will find ways to bend and blend your bodies that will keep you coming back for more. You can employ many tips and tricks to practicing your best sex life. The most important thing to keep in mind is to play safely. I am referring to your hygiene and your use of protection. Taking these issues off the table will allow you to relax into the experience and enjoy your best orgasm. Increase the thrill by leaning a dressing mirror against a wall to watch yourselves play. Enjoy the view of you going down on a mate from the side versus top-down. Light candles, burn incense, create a sexy, romantic, or erotic environment.

Certain positions can serve different purposes. Such as that can be employed to deny orgasm. This is when your mate cannot orgasm until you say so. Some couples who practice BDSM use a strap-on to allow penetrative sex while denying the penis born partner the ability to orgasm.

Double penetration is when you simultaneously penetrate vaginal and anal openings, and aside from using a double-penetration dildo, you can also experience this with a strap-on. A harness is selected that allows the penis to extend under the dildo of the harness, thereby allowing them to insert both the penis and the dildo into the receiver. In the missionary position, the penis would penetrate the anus and the dildo the vagina; in the doggy style, the penis would penetrate the vagina and the dildo the anus. There are harnesses with double penetration toys built in.

You can also find more pleasurable positions when you masturbate. Using non-traditional harnesses, such as furniture attachments and ride-on balls, can be used for masturbation by all genders. A ride-on ball can take the position of another person, in that it can be on bottom for most positions that have the person being penetrated on top, and furniture harnesses can be attached to many objects, an example being a bathtub, to penetrate the user doggy-style.

Here are sex positions that will keep you busy for a little while. Find different variations that fit your needs and keep your sex life fresh and rewarding. Only attempt positions and movement that your healthy enough to perform. Be sure to establish a safe word in case there are any balancing or pressure issues. Of course, this list is not all the joy that can be experienced through exploration and willingness. In respect for all the many ways sex between two or more adults can take place, I am referring to the mates in these positions as the receiver and the giver. Enjoy

MISSIONARY

Raise the receiver's left leg so their knees are level with your right shoulder. Keep the other leg flat on the bed. Thrust toward the inner thigh of the raised leg. This adjustment forces tighter penetration and more clitoral pressure. Receiver could also raise both legs in the air and spread them wider to shorten the vagina around the penis. If you want them deeper, bend your knees and lift them to your chest. Place a pillow under the small of the receiver's back or buttocks to lift the pelvis and change the angle of the penetration. Giver should brace themselves with their hands on the bed in a push up position to take your weight off the receiver's body.

DOGGY STYLE

Doggy style is popular as it is simple, easy, and allows deep thrusting. This position works well for both vaginal and anal penetration and allows deep, smooth strokes; however, it sometimes stimulates the prostate less than other positions during pegging.

THE CAT

Instead of thrusting up and down, rock forward and back to hopefully get enough stimulation for receiver to orgasm. Also, try grinding your pelvis in a circular motion asking receiver to straighten their legs. Receiver should push their pelvis down a few inches while you push up.

MOUNTAIN CLIMBER

Ask him to tease you with a series of moves by entering you with just the tip, thrusting just halfway in then removing himself and stroking you outside with his member. You can reach down and grab his shaft and rub your clitoris with it. Lower yourself to kiss her teasingly while thrusting with your shoulders as well as your pelvis.

QUICKIE FIX

Massage her shoulders to stimulate her breasts by bending over her. Receiver should cross your ankles. This will squeeze your vagina and gluteal muscles tightly around the folic. Reach below to caress her clitoris for extra stimulation.

STANDING TIGER, CROUCHING DRAGON

Make some noise. Explore the deeper sexual response and energy by letting loose with powerful sounds, a roar perhaps. With your legs outside of the receivers, use your thighs to squeeze their knees together, which tighten her vagina around your penis.

WHEELBARROW STANDING

Ask them to rhythmically squeeze her PC muscles to help them climax. You can do this sitting as well. You can also have them walk on her hands as you thrust.

THE BALLET DANCER

Try this standing position in a hot shower. During the steamy foreplay, rub each other's entire body with a coarse salt scrub to stimulate nerve endings and blood flow. If the wrapped leg gets tired, cradle it with your arm; if they are very flexible, lift their leg over your shoulder.

STAND AND DELIVER

Encourage her to play with her clitoris manually. Also, show her that she can control your penetration by flexing her thighs. Have her place her heels on your shoulders, which will open her hips so her labia can press against you.

BUTTER CHURNER

Novelty ignites passion by increasing your brain's levels of dopamine. This position qualifies for novelty, but you don't need to go to such extremes to sustain romance. Participate in this position.

By removing yourself fully, you'll give her the extremely pleasurable feeling of you first entering her repeatedly.

THE FLATIRON

Less friction means less stimulation and can help you last longer. Try using a very slippery silicone-based lubricant which will allow you to thrust longer before reaching orgasm. Receiver, you may be able to increase the intensity of your orgasm by pushing your pelvic floor muscles outward, as if you are trying to squeeze something out of your vagina. This causes your vaginal walls to lower, making your G-spot more accessible. You'll last longer in this position if you switch to shallower thrusts and begin deep breathing. You can also do this on your knees with rear entry but do not thrust deep right away as some find it painful.

THE G-WHIZ

Bring her legs down and have her place her feet on your chest in front of your shoulders. This allows her to control the tempo and depth of thrusts.

THE PRETZEL

Be gentle with her clitoris. It's more sensitive than your penis, so touch lightly at first. Some women even prefer gentle pressure around it rather than direct stimulation. Go soft, then increase speed and pressure and ask her to direct you faster, slower, lighter, harder. Manually stimulate receiver using your fingers. Or withdraw your penis and, holding the shaft with your left hand, rub the head against the clitoris to bring them to the brink of orgasm, then you can reinsert when she wants you inside.

ONE UP

During oral sex, allow the knuckle of your index finger to trail behind your tongue; the contrast between the soft flesh of the tongue and hard bone of the finger will create a pleasing sensation. Let him know the tongue pressure and technique you prefer by demonstrating with your mouth on his earlobe. Encourage her to wriggle a little to help you get the rhythm right. Some women find direct clitoral stimulation uncomfortable. Have her close her legs during oral sex may help. Place your hand above her pubic mound applying light pressure, then rub your firm tongue on the area around the clitoris to add indirect stimulation.

HEIR TO THE THRONE

Insert your index and ring fingers and stroke in a "come hither" motion to wake up the G-spot. With either your tongue or other hand, apply pressure to the pubic bone. This dual stimulation executed just right will send them over the edge. Switch to a swivel chair and turn it left and right as you hold your tongue stationary.

DAVID COPPERFIELD

Let your tongue rest firmly and flat against the full length of her vaginal entrance, then have her move and grind against your tongue. While you lap away, try using your hands to push gently upward on her abdomen, stretching her skin away from her pubic bone and helping to coax the head of her clitoris out from beneath the hood.

THE COWGIRL

It will be easier for her to climax if you stimulate her manually and orally until she is extremely aroused. From the woman-on top position, have her squat over your face where you can orally stimulate her. Give yourself a hand with the V stroke: Make a V with the index and ring finger of one hand and place the fingers on either side of your clitoris with his penis in between. Push your fingers down in a rocking motion. Lie chest to chest on him, stretching your legs out on top of his. Brace your feet on the tops of his and push off to create a rocking motion that will rub your vulva and clitoral area against this pubic bone for greater pleasure.

REVERSE COWGIRL

Lie on your back with legs flat as she straddles you. From this position, you can easily reach down to stimulate yourself or direct the folic to where it feels best. Lean forward or back to change the angle of the folic inside you for greater stimulation.

POLE POSITION

Lie on your back and bend one of your legs up as she sits on you. From Pole position, you can massage his raised leg during the action. Or reach down and touch his perineum. Glance backward to watch him enjoying your erotic movements. Press your vulva hard against his upper thigh, rubbing as the feeling dictates until you reach orgasm.

THE HOT SEAT

Receiver sits in givers lap. From this position they can control the pace and depth of penetration. Plenty of opportunities to be creative in involving all her body. You can reach most of it, include kisses down her back and massage her scalp.

FACE OFF

Ask him to lick your nipples and let his hands roam. There's lots of room for creativity in this face to face straddling position for stimulating erogenous areas of the upper body, head, neck, and face. Sit astride facing him on a rocking chair. Old wooden rockers on hardwood or stone floors provide the greatest variety of good vibes.

THE LAZY MAN

Think of his penis as a masturbatory tool, something to rub and stimulate your clitoris with and against. From this position, you both can lie back into the Spider position or its more challenge variation The X. Simply use the tool as you wish as you control the movement.

SPOON, FACING

Hug each other for 20 seconds before getting busy. Hugging raises your levels of oxytocin, a bonding hormone your body produces naturally, and that will enhance your connection. Because thrusting is more difficult in this position, use different techniques such as grinding, circular, and up and down motions for added stimulation. Use your legs and feet to pull him close during thrusts for deeper penetration as you both lie on your side.

SPORK

Leaning on your arm, slightly tilt your body up on a 45% angle and enter from the side. From the Spork position, you can lift your top leg and support it by resting it on his shoulder. From here, you can easily stimulate your clitoris using your fingers while he is inside you. If you are limber, lift your left leg to increase the depth of penetration.

SPOON

To give her the sensation of greater width inside her, from the Spoon position have her bend and lift her top leg to her breasts. Adjust your position so you are more on top of her top hip than behind her. Lie in front of him facing away from him. He will enter from the rear. You can keep your legs closed or lift the top one in the air. Synchronize your breathing. One of you takes the lead and the other follows so that you inhale and exhale together. The coordinated rhythm opens an unspoken dialogue of intimacy.

THE SPIDER

You can lift her legs onto your shoulders, which increases the muscular tension that advances the orgasm sequence. By elevating your butt off the bed, it'll be easier to thrust and grind in circles. Help him turn you on while he's giving you a massage. Have him straddle your bottom and massage your back. While he's busy with his hands, wiggle, grind and move your mons pubis in a circular motion against the sheets to stimulate your clit. Grab his hands and pull yourself up into a squatting position while he lies back. Or he can remain seated upright and pull you against his chest into the Lazy Man position.

SNOW ANGEL

She lies on her back and you straddle her face down. She will place her legs around your waist and on the back of your shoulders. Grab his butt to help slide up and back and a little massage action to your grip. From this position, you have easy access to fondle his testicles. Lightly run your finger between his testicles and anus to stimulate his perineum. Have him spin around into missionary style to face you while trying to stay inserted. Then switch positions, this time with her on top and facing away.

THE X POSITION

This position could be difficult for some. Once in the position, find a rhythm that works for both of you. Reach out and hold hands to pull together for pelvic thrusting. Also, take turns alternatively sitting up and lying back without changing the rhythm.

THE ELEVATOR

Place a pillow under her head and then straddle her shoulders. Support yourself by holding the bed's headboard or the wall. If your mouth becomes dry after a while, add some mint or fruit flavored lube to his shaft. To keep from gagging when he erupts, you may want to place his penis between your breasts as he nears climax and move it in and out of your cleavage, allowing him to ejaculate over your chest. Don't ignore his balls. Take one of his testicles into your mouth as you stroke his shaft with your hand.

COWGIRL 69

Place a cup of warm tea and an ice cube on the nightstand near the bed. When you give him oral sex, alternate placing the ice cube then the tea in your mouth. Roll over onto your sides in the 69 position. Then massage each other's butts as you lick away.

HOVERING BUTTERFLY

Sit on their face supporting yourself against a wall if needed. Have them hold their tongue firm as you gyrate your hips, pressing your clitoris against it.

SWISS BALL BLITZ

Be careful with this thrilling ride. Balance is necessary as the ball will move and sway with your movements. It's like having sex on a waterbed. Ride the wave of where the ball takes you. Whether it allows you to gyrate or bounce, take advantage of the bounce from the ball.

REST ROOM ATTENDANT

A mirror is sexy. Look at each other in the mirror and share the intimacy of rear entry. Caress all the body parts you can reach. For more control and different angle, place your feet on the toilet seat or tub.

So, you see, there is a rolodex of acts that you can perform alone or with a mate. Remember to only get into positions you can safely move around in. Play safe.

Sexual Health Safety

S afer sex means protecting the health of both you and your sexual partner. Sexual activity and especially sexual intercourse in which various measures (as the use of latex condoms or the practice of monogamy) are taken to avoid disease transmitted by sexual contact. Any tool that can be used to avoid the contraction or spreading of STIs/HIV is practicing safer sex. Myths exist that challenge practicing safer sex. Without modern day sex education, the thought process will always exist.

MYTHS

You Can't Get Pregnant If You're on Top During Vaginal Sex

When a penis born individual has sex with a vulva born individual pregnancy can occur. Cowgirl or any position does not matter. Gravity does not play a role in the route sperm travels. Sex positioning is NOT a form of birth control.

The Pull-Out Method Can Be Used as A Stand-Alone Method of Birth Control

The pull-out (or withdrawal) method, also called coitus interruptus, is when the partner with the penis pulls out of the vagina before ejaculation. This method is only 73% effective according to Planned Parenthood. Using this method with another form of birth control increases effectiveness to 91%.

Men and Women Have "Sexual Peaks" at Different Ages

The word "peak" is a verb described as reaching a highest point, either of a specified value or at a specified time. Alfred C. Kinsey performed a research study in the 20th century that actually counted how many orgasms people of different ages were having. Research has quantified how hormone levels change throughout ones' life and have called the point of the highest level a "peak". There is no data to support that gender has anything to do with your sexual peak. If you perform sex correctly, you can do it if you are physically able to.

Hormonal Birth Control Is Bad for You

"Toxin-free" movements are contributing to birth control myths. It causes weight gain — there is no evidence of this. It can increase your risk for breast cancer — The risk is "slightly increased" but is so small that professionals prescribe it because of its effectiveness. It can prevent pregnancies when you're ready — Once your body resumes non-hormonal regulation, it is highly possible to get pregnant.

Condoms Aren't Effective

Condoms are 98% effective at preventing pregnancy. They are the only method of birth control that also protects against most sexually transmitted infections (STIs). Size does matter. Don't go magnum when basic will do. The wrong size will prevent the condom from doing its job. You CANNOT reuse condoms.

There's No Male Birth Control

Men can employ birth control methods. A true pill is in the works and research gets closer every day. Men are responsible for using a condom. Every time.

A Person with A Penis Can't Enjoy Sex While Wearing A Condom

Ask the question, if sex with a condom feels like nothing, how is orgasm possible? Men express to women that the feeling with a condom desensitizes the pleasure. Guilt over his orgasm should not be a reason to not use a condom.

You Can't Get Pregnant If You Have Sex in Water

You cannot wash sperm out of the vagina to avoid pregnancy. Sex in water does not prevent your exposure to STI/Ds. Once sperm enters the uterus, there is nothing you can do to reverse it. Water does not prevent sperm from traveling its natural course.

Masturbation Makes Achieving Orgasm More Difficult

Note that vulva owners can numb their genitals with too much vibration. If you don't know what makes you cum, how can you expect your partner to figure it out? Using toys is a great way to increase pleasure in masturbating.

Having A Lot of Sex Is Shameful

Slut-shaming. Safer Sex with multiple partners. There is nothing shameful about enjoying a lot of sex. Prioritize safety, consent, and pleasure and have as much sex as wanted.

You Can't Get STIs from Oral Sex

STI/Ds CAN be transmitted through oral sex for all partners. You can spread, Chlamydia, Trichomoniasis, Gonorrhea, Herpes,

HPV, Syphilis and HIV during oral sex. Transferrable via saliva, mouth cuts, or sores. Use condoms or dental dams to create a barrier between partners.

If You Have A Lot of Sex, Your Vagina Will Get "Loose"

Vaginal muscle tissue is very elastic and no folic is going to make it "looser". Differentiate the muscles that exist in the vagina. There is no normal when it comes to vaginas; loose is subjective.

Anal Doesn't Count as Sex

Anal is a sex act. Anal has become more acceptable among many genders. Shame is the largest reason for this myth. Anal sex exposes individuals to STI/Ds.

Lesbians Don't Get STIs

Different sex acts carry different risks. The risk of spreading STIs is also higher if there's a lot of friction. STI risk is higher when you or one of your partners is on their period. Exposure can happen during any of the following: Unprotected oral sex Manual sex (fingering) Sharing sex toys, Using a strap-on, Tribbing, Analingus

Taking the Pill Means I Practice Safe Sex

The pill is birth control but not a barrier for STI/Ds. Women who believe this myth increase their chances of contracting an STI/D by 100%. Safer sex must include a barrier for all sex acts.

Menstruation Is the Ultimate Baby Barrier

There is a chance that you can get pregnant during your menses. Understand that the average cycle last 28 days. You must know where in the cycle you are after period sex. 3-5 days of the 28-day cycle is when you are voiding unfertilized eggs. Women are most fertile during the ovulation state of the menstrual cycle.

Drinking and Drugs Make Sex Much More Fun

This is dangerous, but it may seem true. You are less likely to practice safe sex. Your ability to give consent is lowered. Substance use can cause impotence, premature ejaculation, inability to orgasm and other side effects.

TV And Movies Portray Sex as It Really Is

TV is entertainment, not sex education. In entertainment, there is no talk about STIs prior to sex acts. Most of what you see will never happen in real life. Sex as it really is, includes safe sex conversations.

These myths are detrimental to our sexual health. We are not going to be able to eradicate sexually transmitted viruses without modern-day sex education. Not enough people are practicing safe sex and thus, viruses that we have been discussing and treating for generations still exist. Each year the patients are getting younger and younger. This is why I do what I do. There are some viruses that we should not be talking about today; if I can teach one individual to live a healthier sex life, I have met my mark.

Sexually Transmitted Infections and Diseases

TRICHOMONIASIS (TRICH)

Trichomoniasis is a common sexually transmitted disease that affects both men and women. Trichomoniasis is caused by a protozoan parasite called Trichomonas vaginalis and is a cause of vaginal infections and urethral infections in penis born individuals. Trichomoniasis is spread through sexual contact. Transmission can occur even if a person does not have symptoms of infection. Women contract trichomoniasis from infected male or female partners, while men usually contract it only from female partners. Using condoms and/or dental dams provide some protection. Their use is strongly encouraged but is not 100% safe.

Trichomoniasis is one of the most common and most curable STD's. The symptoms are more annoying than they are threatening to your health. The genital inflammation caused by trichomoniasis might however, increase a person's risk of acquiring HIV infection if they are exposed to HIV or might also increase the chances of transmitting HIV infection to a sex partner. In rare cases, trichomoniasis in pregnant women may cause a premature rupture of the membranes and early delivery.

SCABIES

Some physicians do not consider scabies as an STI; however, because it is highly contagious and spreads from skin to skin contact, it is considered an STI by the CDC. It spreads very fast in crowded areas when close body contact is frequent as well as during personal contact. Nowadays, dermatologists can easily diagnose and successfully treat scabies.

Scabies is an infestation, not an infection. Tiny mites reproduce on the skin surface, burrow in the outer layers of the skin, and plant eggs in there. This skin condition is characterized by intense itching and skin rash. The mite is often spread during skin-to-skin contact with a person who is already infested with scabies. The skin rash looks typical for some other diseases too, so scabies may be easily confused with other conditions in its early stages. For example, acne and mosquito bites can look like scabies. What sets the latter apart is severe itching. Each year millions of people contract scabies all over the world. The young people and the old are two groups commonly affected by scabies.

Scabies mites can be present at any area of the body, but their favorite places include warm spots between fingers, around breast creases and the buttock, under fingernails, around the navel and waistline, or within skin folds. They also hide under bracelets, rings or watch straps.

Scabies mites cannot fly or jump; they crawl slowly instead, so the only way for them to move from one person to another is to wait for the people to have extended physical contact. Holding hands can transmit scabies, but typically it is not spread through a hug or a quick handshake. The disease can be quickly passed between sexual partners or household members. Shared personal items may be to blame if they are contaminated. Scabies parasites can survive outside the body for 24 to 36 hours. Scabies can be contracted through wearing clothes or sleeping in bedding that is infested. After a person has been infested for the first time, symptoms may show up in around 4–6 weeks. The symptoms develop more quickly in those people who have already had scabies before. If it's a recurrence, symptoms appear in 1–4 days after the exposure. Once infested, a person is contagious and can pass scabies to other people even if they have not developed any symptoms yet.

SYPHILIS

Syphilis belongs to a group of infections which are transmitted sexually. The first stage of infection development involves genitals' sores, which are not accompanied by any painful feelings. If not treated, the infection can develop throughout many years, which can lead to rather harmful consequences to other parts of the body. It can have a negative impact on human's heart and brain. At the same time, syphilis can be treated rather easily and fast without any bad consequences for patient's health on its early stages. It is rather important for your partner also to be examined if syphilis was diagnosed. It is caused by a special type of germ called Treponema pallidum. It is one of the most common sexually transmitted diseases. The number of infected patients is increasing from year to year.

The incubation period is one week to three months. Through oral, anal, or vaginal sex, via intimate touching or kissing. Some people mistakenly think that infection can be obtained via toilet seats, bathtubs, shared clothing, etc. This is a false opinion. Syphilis can be obtained only via direct contact with a person who already has the infection. Infection can be also transmitted via blood. It can be brought to human's organism with the help of blood receiving a transfusion. That is why it is important to proceed with thorough and accurate examination of blood receiving products. Needle sharing between infected patients can also result in syphilis.

HEPATITIS A-E

There are five types of hepatitis, A through E, all of which cause liver inflammation. Type D affects only those who also have hepatitis B, and hepatitis E is extremely rare in the US. Type A hepatitis is contracted through anal-oral contact, by coming in contact with the feces of someone with hepatitis A, or by eating or drinking hepatitis A contaminated food or water. Type B hepatitis can be contracted from infected blood, seminal fluid, vaginal secretions, or contaminated drug needles, including tattoo or body-piercing equipment. Type C hepatitis is not easily spread through sex. You're more likely to get it through contact with infected blood, contaminated razors, needles, tattoo and body-piercing equipment, or manicure or pedicure tools that haven't been properly sanitized, and a mother can pass it to her baby during delivery.

Type D hepatitis can be passed through contact with infected blood, contaminated needles, or by sexual contact with an HIV-infected person. Type E hepatitis is most likely to be transmitted in feces, through oral contact, or in water that's been contaminated. The incubation period is between two weeks to five months, although Type C can remain dormant for 10 years before symptoms crop up. If you are not treated, because types A and E usually go away over time, neither is likely to lead to chronic disease. Types B and C, however, can lead to cirrhosis (scarring of the liver) and liver cancer if not treated; type D can also result in liver cancer.

MOLLUSCUM CONTAGIOSUM

Although the virus can affect anyone, there are some specific conditions when a person becomes an easy target for the virus. People who are more likely to get this virus include children aged between 1 and 10, people with weak immune system (those with AIDS or having chemotherapy, steroid or cancer treatment), people having atopic dermatitis, people having skin-to-skin contact with the infected person The virus is contagious. It usually spreads through skin-to-skin contact that includes sexual contact or touching the bumps.

Molluscum Contagiosum not only spreads from one person to another but also from one part of the body to the other parts. You can spread the virus in your body by touching, scratching, or squeezing the spots. The thick yellowy-white substance, when released after the bump has been ruptured, is highly infectious.

PUBIC LICE

Also known as crabs, they are often found around the genitals; they can live in any part of the body with hair. Crabs are usually transmitted via close contact with an infected person including sex. It is commonly followed by various symptoms and side effects such as itching. If crab disease has been diagnosed, patients need complete STD treatment course which involves insecticide creams and lotions which help to terminate the lice.

Crabs are contracted through sexual transmission, skin-to-skin contact or through clothing, bedding and toilet seat harboring the insects. Contracting lice can be divided into two main classifications. They include pubic lice and body lice. Every type of lice can be contracted in several ways. Pubic lice can be passed from one person to another after close contact. The most common way is having sex with infected person. At the same time there are several non-sexual ways to catch lice.

Various physical contacts may also be the reason for infection. They include kissing a person who has lice in his beard, for example. Pay attention that pubic lice can attach strongly to your pubic hairs. It will be quite hard to wash them out using common methods. They will not fall out by themselves. The fact that genital crabs call for their host to feed on, you are very unlikely to obtain lice from clothes, shared towels, bed lined or toilet seats. Crabs' incubation period is as long as a week if it's the first time you've had pubic lice as little as a day if this is a recurrence.

HPV (HUMAN PAPILLOMA VIRUS

Human Papillomavirus, is commonly referred to as HPV, is a vast group of viruses potentially leading to genital warts and, in worst cases, cancer. However, most HPV types do not harm the human body, go away in several months and remain unnoticed. Sexually active people are more likely to obtain the infection, and more than a half of all people acquire it over the course of life.

Human Papillomavirus is a sexually transmitted disease as it is normally transmitted during sexual contact. There is no direct medicine to cure Human Papillomavirus. However, there are vaccines to prevent you from getting dangerous types of the virus and simple guidelines that can help you stay clear of the disease. If you have contracted the virus, there are several ways, including surgical, to get rid of the symptoms, such as warts. Serious cases, including cancer, need to have a complex medical approach. HPV A, E and D typically go away on their own and do not require special treatment.

It is difficult to determine the average period of time required for the virus to go away from the body as it is usually unclear when it has been contracted. However, it can take as much as several years for the virus' symptoms to go away after the moment they have been detected. Human Papillomavirus stands for the large group of easily transmitted viruses that potentially can cause cancer. They are usually transmitted during sexual intercourse, including oral, vaginal, anal sex and other skin-to-skin contacts. However, the infection can also enter someone's body through any natural fluids or even minor skin cuts. HPV is one of the most spread sexually transmitted diseases.

HIV AND AIDS

HIV is the acronym for the Human Immunodeficiency Virus, a virus that attacks the body's immune system, leading to full-blown AIDS (Acquired Immunodeficiency Syndrome). AIDS is devastating because it leaves the body susceptible to life-threatening infections and certain kinds of cancers.

It is transmitted through oral, anal, or vaginal sex and from an HIV-positive mother to her baby. To prevent it, use a condom every time you have sex; find out the sexual history of any new partners, including their HIV status; and don't share needles if you do intravenous drugs.

The incubation period is varied as some people develop symptoms shortly after being infected, but it takes more than ten years for symptoms to appear for many. If you are not treated, HIV progresses more rapidly into full-blown AIDS without treatment, usually because of infections that develop because of the patient's weakened immune system.

GONORRHEA (THE CLAP)

Gonorrhea is a highly contagious sexually transmitted bacterial infection, sometimes referred to as "the clap". The nickname of the clap refers to a treatment that used to clear the blockage in the urethra from gonorrhea pus, where the penis would be 'clapped' on both sides simultaneously. This treatment is rarely used today; however, the nomenclature remains. Gonorrhea is characterized by thick discharge from the penis or vagina.

Gonorrhea spreads through semen or vaginal fluids during unprotected sexual contact with an infected partner: Vaginal or anal sex with an infected partner, oral sex, although this is less common sharing sex toys touching parts of the body with fingers (for example, touching the genitals and then the eyes) any very close physical contact. The bacteria can be passed from hand to hand in very rare isolated cases, from a mother to her baby at birth You can NOT catch it from simple kissing, sharing baths, towels, cups, or from toilet seats. It incubates in 1–14 days from exposure.

If not treated, Gonorrhea infection can spread through the bloodstream to other parts of the body, causing damage and serious problems. In women, it can cause life-threatening complications such as ectopic pregnancy (outside the womb) blocked fallopian tubes (the tubes which carry the egg from the ovaries to the womb), which can result in reduced fertility or infertility long-term pelvic pain. In men, it can lead to painful inflammation of the testicles, which may result in reduced fertility or sterility

HERPES

There are two types of viral infections characterized by periodic outbreaks of painful sores. Stress, sunburn, sex, and certain foods are the primary causes of a herpes outbreak.

Both herpes simplex virus-1 and virus-2 may be transmitted through sex or by kissing or touching any affected area. A condom can prevent herpes transmission during vaginal or anal sex, but oral contact with genitals or open sores anywhere can spread the disease.

Washing hands can also minimize transmission. The incubation period is anywhere from five to twenty days.

If you are not treated, while herpes is not life-threatening, and not all people who have it suffer from outbreaks, it can lead to other health problems.

VAGINAL YEAST

A naturally occurring fungus called Candida albicans (C. Albicans) usually causes this type of vaginitis. Many of you probably know vaginal yeast infection as candidiasis. It is an absolutely normal condition for women. It is named so because vaginal yeast infection can be caused by fungus candida. It is usually followed by several unpleasant side effects, including swelling, irritation and itching.

The latest medical research shows that 3 out of 4 women may get vaginal yeast infection at a point in their lives regardless of age. In addition, women are very likely to have more infections in future. It usually occurs more than once.

The infection spread by various ways, including sexual contact. Patients will hardly face any difficulties in treating vaginal yeast infections. Still, it will depend on the level of disease severity, The incubation period anywhere from 12 hours to five days.

If you are not treated, vaginal yeast infections don't cause serious complications. If it is not treated, the itching may persist. At the same time, if traditional treatment did not come in handy, you can also try several popular alternative methods. On the one hand, it will make it possible to avoid taking prescribed drugs; on the other you can do it at home without visiting your doctor. Common alternative methods include using vinegar douches or garlic; yogurt or tea tree oil cream inserted into the vagina.

VAGINOSIS (BV)

Bacterial vaginosis (BV) is a widely spread health problem which results in vaginal discharge. Sexual activity can cause vaginosis. Such overgrowth can lead to common BV symptoms which are rather mild in most cases. Luckily for patients, they will not face any difficulties in clearing BV without taking medications. But in some cases, more efficient treatment may be necessary. Bacterial vaginosis (BV) results from overgrowth of one of several organisms that are normally present in vagina, upsetting the natural balance of vaginal bacteria. More than one in six women in the United States has bacterial vaginosis, though many aren't aware of having it.

BV has nothing in common with any other complicated infections. It is rather simple and is caused by simple germs. Under normal conditions, vagina contains a mixture of bacteria. When BV occurs, balance changes. Specialists still do not know the exact reason why this happens. The result is that some bacteria start multiplying more actively.

Intensive washing of the vagina can also lead to bacteria unbalance altering and creating perfect environment for BV progressing. This type of vaginitis can spread during sexual intercourse, but it also happens to people who aren't sexually active. Females with new or multiple sex partners, as well as females who use an intrauterine device (IUD) for birth control, have a higher risk of obtaining bacterial vaginosis. Despite all known reasons of BV contraction there are still lots of arguments about the fact how infections get to the organism or how common it may be. This is because infection is commonly rather mild and there is no necessity to consult the doctor.

If you are not treated, Bacterial vaginosis is usually not serious. In some cases, however, it can cause infections in the uterus and fallopian tubes. It is important to treat bacterial vaginosis, especially before having an IUD inserted, an abortion, or tests done on the uterine lining. Both trichomoniasis and bacterial vaginosis have been linked to an increased risk of transmission of human immunodeficiency virus (HIV) and other sexually transmitted diseases.

Unfortunately, there is no reliable way to avoid BV occurrence in the future. It is hard to prevent due to its natural origin and development. The vagina does not need any specific cleaning. It means that you should avoid pushing water into it; avoid using too much bath oil, scented soap, bubbles, antiseptics, and other substances while taking a bath; avoid using powerful detergents while washing your underwear; avoid washing zones around the vulva and vagina very often. You may proceed with washing once a day. The incubation period is anywhere from 12 hours to five days.

YEAST IN MEN (BALANITIS)

Balanitis, yeast infection in men, can get yeast infection of the genitals. Yeast organisms are a common cause of infection of the tip of the penis, a condition called Balanitis. Balanitis can be described as inflammation of the penis glans. It can also result in foreskin inflammation which covers the head of penis unless the male was circumcised. But sometimes, both foreskin and glans can be damaged at the same time.

The main problem about this disease is the fact that it can occur at any age. At the same time, Balanitis is more likely to affect a male under 4 years old. It can also be observed with adult men who avoided circumcising. According to the latest statistics, 1 of 25 boys under 4 may suffer from this unpleasant inflammation. At the same time, Balanitis affects every thirtieth man who has not been circumcised. There are several types of Balanitis causes. They include non-infection and infection causes. The disease can mainly be found in patients who have too tight foreskin of their penises. In addition, males who suffer from diabetes are also prone to such inflammation. Moreover, in this case, Balanitis can develop rapidly.

Causes of Balanitis Disease can result in various health problems including balanitis xerotica obliterans. It refers to chronic dermatitis, which involves damaging not only of foreskin but also the glans. Phimosis is also included in the list of possible consequences. It mainly occurs when the foreskin is very tight. Paraphimosis is another common problem when a patient can't return the foreskin to the original location after it was retracted. Cancer is probably the most severe possible consequence.

One is more likely to get Balanitis if they are uncircumcised or have diabetes. It should also be noted that most men do not have the foggiest idea that they have yeast infection. It can be in progress without any notice. Infection is mainly contracted from the males' partners. Men may be unable to identify its symptoms for a certain period which can lead to yeast development. Therefore, it is common when they are simply informed about the fact by their partners. Another way to identify infection is to complete a medical examination as soon as possible. They may start feeling certain discomfort and irritation in some occasions. That is why it is rather important to be well-aware of all possible symptoms to prevent disease development at short notice without harmful consequences. The incubation period may vary from 12 hours to 5 days.

PELVIC INFLAMMATORY DISEASE (PID)

Pelvic Inflammatory Disease (PID) is an infection affecting the female reproductive organs. PID typically comes as a complication of various sexually transmitted diseases, mainly caused by Chlamydia or Gonorrhea bacteria. Responsible for over 90% of all cases. When left untreated, PID can lead to serious, often irreversible damage to the female reproductive system, namely uterus, ovaries, and fallopian tubes.

Untreated PID is the most common reason for female infertility that can be prevented. Every year over a million women in the UIS alone fall into an episode of PID. Consequently, more than 100,000 of them face infertility every year. Apart from that, PID is responsible for a large amount of ectopic pregnancies. Abortion, childbirth, and other pelvic operations are among other causes. In a healthy body, the cervix prevents bacteria from entering the internal reproductive organs from the vagina. However, when exposed to sexually transmitted diseases, the cervix gets infected and loses its protective functions, allowing the infections and bacteria to reach the upper genital tract and reproductive organs.

Being mainly caused by other sexually transmitted diseases, PID is easily transmitted if a person is exposed to risk factors and follows controversial sexual behavior. Here are the factors that make women susceptible to Pelvic Inflammatory Disease: having several sexual partners; having an untrustworthy sexual partner who might have other contacts rather than you; having had PID before; being a sexually active young person, particularly under 25; douching might help bacteria enter the upper genital organs and hide any sorts of uncommon discharge that could help diagnose an infection; using an IUD for the purpose of birth control.

CHLAMYDIA

Chlamydia is a common curable bacterial sexually transmitted disease (STD). Chlamydia trachomatis, or simply chlamydia, is an infection caused by pathogen bacterium that can afflict the cervix in females and the urethra and rectum in both males and females. Occasionally other parts of the body, such as the lining of the eyelid, throat, and rectum, can be affected. Untreated Chlamydia can lead to cystitis, inflammation of the urinary bladder, an inflammation of the cervix with yellowish vaginal discharge and pain during sexual intercourse. In males, untreated chlamydia can lead to painful inflammation of the inner structures of the testicles, which may cause reduced fertility or sterility.

A rare complication of Epididymitis is as well, reactive arthritis, which causes pain in the inflamed joints that can be disabling prostatitis occasionally, Reiter's syndrome (arthritis, inflammation of urethra and eyes) Urethritis, inflammation of the urethra, with a yellow discharge appearing at the tip of the penis. Untreated urethritis results in narrowing of the urethra which leads to painful urinating and can cause kidney problems.

More than 90 million cases of Chlamydia are reported each year globally with more than a half occurring in females. The highest rate of infections is observed among teens and young adults. About half of men and most women infected with chlamydia trachomatis do not observe any symptoms, which leads to the disease being untreated and easily passed from partner to partner. Chlamydia can be cured easily with simple antibiotics otherwise; serious complications can occur in the reproductive system such as PID and even infertility.

Chlamydia is transmitted primarily through sexual activity. The following are the most common ways to contract Chlamydia: unprotected intercourse (vaginal, anal) with an infected partner oral sex, although a less common cause of infection as bacteria Chlamydia trachomatis targets the genital area rather than the throat. Although it is possible theoretically, the cases of infestation from mouth-to-penis and penis-to-mouth contact are rare. Vagina, cervix, anus, penis, or mouth contacting infected secretions or fluids which means that contraction can occur even if the penis or tongue does not enter the vagina or anus.

Bacteria can travel from the vaginal area to the anus or rectum of females while wiping with toilet paper sharing sex toys, from mother to the newborn during vaginal childbirth through the infected birth canal. Infection can be transferred on fingers from the genitals to other parts of the body (for example, chlamydia can occur in the eyes) Chlamydia is not contracted through simple kissing, hand-shaking, any casual contacts, sharing baths, towels and cups as well as from toilet seats. The incubation period of Chlamydia is 7–21 days.

HPV (WARTS)

Human Papilloma Virus (HPV) — a group of more than 70 viruses, several strains of HPV cause external genital warts. It is contracted through oral, anal, and vaginal sex and through skin-to-skin contact. The incubation period is anywhere from one month to several years.

If you are not treated and genital warts are allowed to grow without treatment, they can block the vagina, urethra, or anus and become very uncomfortable. Depending on where they are on the body, genital warts can cause sores and bleeding. An increase in the size and number of the warts is also more likely during pregnancy and when a person's immune system is compromised by diabetes, an organ transplant, Hodgkin's disease, or HIV/AIDS, among other conditions.

Keeping it Sexy

You are deep into a long-term relationship and the lust is dulling. There is something you can do about that. Learn to set yourself up for success. Feeling good about yourself will help you to be able to give to your sexual relationships.

THINGS TO DO

- Show your style.

- Look in the mirror. Pick your features of which you are most satisfied with, and show them off with clothes, makeup, or accessories. If you seem to know what you've got, others will get the message and notice you for what you have.

- Invest in a good pair of curve-hugging jeans. Dark denim looks good on all body types.

- Pick some clothes that flatter your figure and that you feel comfortable in. There's no point picking the latest fashions if you don't feel comfortable in them. Pick clothes that make you feel like you.

- Wear lace-up flats or sneakers. Flats are cute and comfortable, two characteristics that you rarely ever find together in the shoe department.

- Wear jewelry that excites you. Find colorful, fun, bright chunky necklaces, and bracelets, but if you wear lots of pearls and beads, don't wear a shirt that has a pattern or a picture on it. Wear a monochromatic top with lots of multi-colored jewelry.

- Black is sexy. It hides fat, creates curves, and makes you feel like a goddess.

- Sexy undergarments. But don't flash them. Be classy about it otherwise, you look trashy. Try to maintain class as much as possible while still being sexy.

- Take up dancing. Sign up for dance lessons with a friend, salsa, ballet, hip-hop, ballroom, whatever you like. You'll gain confidence, and you will move more gracefully and sexily in everything you do, without even thinking about it. Health benefits are an obvious bonus. Belly dancing is also another way to feel sexy and confident.

- Wear make-up. Just make sure not to go overboard. Subtle is very sexy in the same way that less is more. Accent one feature at a time. For example, one day, put on lip-liner, bold red lipstick, and mascara. For another day, wear subtle pink or clear lip gloss, and wear eyeliner to make your eyes stand out. If you need help creating a look, a mall makeup counter or independent beauty consultant would be happy to teach you for free.

- If you're dissatisfied with your body, by all means, work on getting healthier, but remember that "sexy" isn't a body shape. It's an aura. So, start working on feeling sexy now. Getting slim and toned can augment sexiness, but it can never replace it. Owning a Steinway isn't the same thing as being a master pianist; in the same way, owning a "hot" body isn't the same thing as being sexy. Learn to play the "piano" you've got. Work it and love it and everyone else will too.

- Sexy doesn't equal skinny. Men are attracted to all body types. Curvy women are sexy too.

- Also remember, confidence is the key. Sex appeal involves a belief in yourself that you can and will appear sexy. Most public icons or even film stars carry their sexiness in their confidence. Even a simple smile shows confidence and appeal. In fact, the starting point to sexiness starts with confidence.

- Touching or licking your lips draws attention and looks really sexy; if they like you, they will immediately think about kissing you.

- If you feel sexy and confident, then it will show, occasionally raise your eyebrows, and flutter those eyelashes.

- Highlight your positive features. If you have pretty blue eyes, then show them off. If you have a beautiful smile, then flash those pearly whites.

- Show a little bit of cleavage if you are older. Make sure you look classy, subtle, and appropriate.

- Drink lots of water and eat nutritious food. Be healthy. Curves are sexy. If you are naturally slim, this is also lovely.

- Wear pretty lingerie and underwear, even if no one sees it.

- Wear nail polish. For example, clear polish on fingernails and bright red and hot pink on toenails.

- Look to others for inspiration...for example Beyoncé, Marilyn Monroe, Natalie Wood, and Sophia Loren.

- Find your passion in life. Do you love to dance? Act? Sing?

- Listen to music that makes you move your hips

16 DAYS AND DOZENS OF WAYS TO REIGNITE ROMANTIC LOVE

Day 1: Appreciate How Good You've Got It

Keep your eye on your prize and know that finding someone new, divorce and affairs sound easier than they really are.

- Grab a pad and list all the things you like about your mate

- Write down memorable things you have done together.

- Reflect on all the ways you are better off with this person in your life.

- Review your list every day for 2 weeks.

Day 2: Tell a Secret

If you have an affair or other such secret tell. Sometimes the honesty can help towards working through the infidelities. Don't Lie.

- It fosters a deeper level of intimacy that leads to a more lasting trust.

- It allows your relationship to keep pace with the changes occurring in each of you.

- It keeps channels of communication open and provides constant challenges that can be used for growth.

- It allows each of you to know yourselves at even deeper levels and use all your resources to build the best relationship possible.

Day 3: Learn Their Language

Things that make you feel great may not be the things that make them feel great. Learn the language that makes your spouse weak in the knees.

- I feel especially loved when someone expresses how grateful they are for me and the simple things I do.

- I feel especially loved when a person gives me undivided attention and spends time alone with me.

- I feel especially loved by someone who brings me gifts and other tangible expressions of love.

- I feel especially loved when someone pitches in to help me, perhaps by running errands or taking on my household chores.

- I feel especially loved when a person expresses feelings for me through physical contact.

- Spend the rest of the week focuses on meeting your partner's top two love needs.

Day 4: Put Sex on the Calendar

Beyond V-day and birthdays, make sex a priority.

- Pick other holidays

- Pick other locations

- Determine which outdoor places or locations can be thrilling for you both.

Day 5: Start Foreplay at 6:30 a.m.

Foreplay can take place PRIOR to the 3 minutes before insertion.

- Start the day with a long embrace.

- Send a dirty text message, note under the windshield.

- Call her in the middle of the day to ask how SHE is doing.

Day 6: Use the Whole Field

Utilize all of the square footage of your home for sex. Not just the bedroom.

- Living Room — Use the coffee table the night before a party or dinner. Keep her secretly smiling throughout the event.

- Laundry — On the washer or dryer during the spin cycle. You can do penetration with her legs on shoulders or perform oral.

- Bathroom — Have her hold onto the sink as you enter from the back. The mirror eye contact in this position is instant intimacy.

- Stairs — Sit on the stairs facing the railing, have her sit in your lap and take an unexpected ride.

- Sofa — Have her straddle the arm of the sofa facedown, use a scarf under her so that her mound and clit rub against it as you thrust.

- Outdoors — Cool breeze on naked skin, smells, sounds and fear of getting caught makes this a must-do.

Day 7: Be Assertive, Not Insertive.

This is sexual contact without penetration. VENIS = Very Erotic Non-Insertive Sex.

- Have one night when intercourse isn't the focus.

Day 8: Have Morning Sex

It makes you feel bonded all day long.

- Get Fresh: Sneaking off to brush your teeth will add intimacy.

- Get Cozy: Get a position that takes little to know effort. You can do a lying rear entry taking advantage of your free hands.

Day 9: Control Anger.

Screaming matches are poor foreplay.

- Control major outburst of anger.

- Don't take everything personal and allow for some mood adjustments.

- The conversation should be constructive and proves how much each partner values the other's opinions.

- Fight or flight adrenaline will drive you further into an angry, defensive response.

Day 10: Enjoy a Quickie

Women don't always need 10 or 20 minutes of foreplay.

- Heart-pounding adrenaline of spontaneous sex can be a huge erotic rush.

- Dry Hump on the sofa until she is reaching for your zipper.

- Engage in a seductive long kiss while cooking dinner. Lean her against a cabinet and as she melts in your arms, lift her skirt, or pull off her pants while sitting her on the counter. This is not rough, its deliberate and a huge turn on.

Day 11: Scare Your Pants Off

Get risky, then get frisky.

- Trying something new before sex delivers a burst of dopamine that activates pleasure.

Day 12: Knead Each Other

A massage is intimacy and pleasure even if it does not lead to sex.

- Use an oil, massager, or your warmed hands.

- Stroke toward the heart. When working on her legs, stroke upward. On the arms, stroke downward.

- Ease with effleurage. Effleurage is a simple loosen-up stroke. Light, long and rhythmic running with the grain of the muscle. On the legs, use your cupped palms and gently glide upward. On the back, flatten your hands and broaden your strokes.

- Play with petrissage. Circular stroke designed to squeeze the muscles and wring out tension from the shoulders, upper arms, legs, and buttocks. Use both hands to work the muscles in opposite directions. Move one palm away from you as you slide it forward and move the other toward you.

- Roll your thumbs. Best for working on tension knots. Use your thumbs one after the other to press into the flesh.

Sometimes moving circularly and other times just holding pressure on the point. Lean your weight into it.

- Be generous. Don't forget the body parts that rarely get touched, such as the backs of the arms, and knees, feet, fingers, and scalp.

Day 13: Watch Porn or an Erotic Film Together

Watching other people have sex can trigger lusty thoughts about your partner and spice up your sex life.

- Have a heart to heart talk about how they really feel about erotic movies and porn in general.

- Pick films in which the actors look more physically like you or your partner so that the body types are ones that turn you on.

- Try to reenact what you saw.

Day 14: Become a Stranger

We sometimes get different after we marry.

- Write down a list of 10 things you did pre-marriage. How many related to your core being are you still doing?

- Fill up the tires on your old road bike? Golf or take a river run to reinvent yourself.

- Becoming who you were may be strange to her and start the connection all over again.

- The sex gets better over time is an old rule. Now the sex gets better over time if you help it get better.

- Give room and opportunities for your mate to revert or make changes to their personalities.

Day 15: Employ Some Toys

Cock Rings, vibrators, dildos, or pumps can enhance the entire experience.

- The Classic Dildo. Most women concentrate on their clit, penetrating only when ready to climax. Thus, use your penis to stroke the outer labia and clit during foreplay. Gyrating along with these pleasure points by increasing pressure will push her desire to the tipping point so that when you penetrate, you will deliver an orgasm-inducing thrust.

- The G-Spot Stimulator. These toys target the spongy, sensitive area in her upper vaginal wall. A G-Spot orgasm comes from strategic pressure not size. Thus, use your penis to add pressure with each thrust, enter her when she is on her back with her knees resting on her chest.

- The Rabbit Vibrator. This hare looking toy rubs both sides of her clitoris. Thus, use your index and ring fingers to rub the sides. Simultaneously stroke the top of her clit with a middle finger, completing the trick to send her over the edge.

- The Classic Vibrator. Multispeed massage that lets her focus on nerve-rich erogenous spot, the clitoris, as it intensifies. Thus, a little change is good. Start slow, gentile, and use broad strokes with your finger and tongue. Build toward a climax, instead of rapidly changing techniques and intensity.

Day 16: Turn Them on in the Kitchen

Make dinner and doing the dishes afterward.

- Recognize all they do and give her a well-deserved break.

- Eliminate stresses that stifle their sexual thoughts and motivation.

- Womyn are not interested in sex when they are stressed, tired, and distracted. This is a fact.

- Use touch without a sexual motive to endorse her, a caress, a kiss, a tender tap.

There truly are some very creative ways you can keep the lust alive in a long-term relationship. You in fact can use all the techniques, tips, and information in this book to build a sexual plan that will keep you safe and healthy, and pleasantly sexually fulfilled.

Well there you have it. A ton of information that you can use to create your most fulfilling orgasm. Use this book to practice and explore and become an orgasm master. There is a lot of modern-day sex education topics that can open the door to better sex. When you realize the power of great sex, you will find yourself living a healthier more fulfilling life. The benefits of orgasm are vast and can change your life. Realize the power you hold and begin to explore it and own it.

References

Andrews, T., Hsieh, C., May 23, 2019, 22 Hot Spots on a Man's Body You Should Definitely Know About. Retrieved March 19, 2020, from: https://www.cosmopolitan.com/sex-love/a2299/9-triggers/

Barnes, Vickie June 28, 2019, How Does the Cervix Change at Ovulation? https://www.babyhopes.com/blogs/fertility/cervix-change

Healio Health. 2019. Retrieved September 5, 2019, from: https://healiohealth.com/products/index/1630

Mitra Samar, June 1, 2015 Anatomy: Part 1 7th Edition Academic Publishers page 460–480.

Rimm, H., December 11, 2017, 5 Types of Orgasms and How to Get One (or More) Retrieved September 3, 2019 from: https://www.healthline.com/health/healthy-sex/types-of-orgasms

WebMd. 2019 Painful Sex in Women. Retrieved October 14, 2019, from: https://www.webmd.com/sexual-conditions/guide/female-pain-during=sex#2

Weston, L., March/April 2018 Can't Orgasm? Here's Help for Women. Retrieved September 3, 2019, from:
https://www.webmd.com/sexual-conditions/features/cant-orgasm-heres-help-for-women#1

About the Author

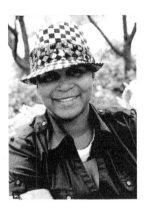

Debra Shade is a Clinical Sexologist and Master Sexpert, with many varied accomplishments in the adult industry. She runs a private practice working with couples and individuals of all genders and orientations. She is IMBd accredited for the alternative TV series "Web Cam Diaries" presently in pre-production for After Hours HD on Roku TV, and is the author of three intensely erotic books, *Maybe She is Right, Hot Sex on a Platter* and *Queen B.*

She possesses an unmistakable charisma in her educational approach, she transcends the convention of "workshops," and provides each participant with an encounter that offers personalized instruction with hands-on physical technique applications. Shade assists individuals and couples to help them break through barriers to their best sexual experiences. She works at reconnecting relationships, teaching how to orgasm and empower clients with tools and techniques to ensure their best sexual experience.

Shade delivers workshops and seminars on modern day sex education in various settings. Known for pushing the envelope, she currently hosts adult sex education conversations titled "Sexy Talk and Play" which is an engaging happy hour and learning experience. She is also host of "Adult Recess," "BLISS," "'Womyn4Womyn," "Sip & Paint Nudes," "High Rise," "Shade's Oasis," "Revelry" and "Aphrodisia."

Debra is also called upon to provide experiences for private parties in need of a Sexpert. She has delivered for expos, conventions and festivals, such as the 2019 National Sexual Health Conference, The Ohio Lesbian Festival, TRAUMA, Lion's Den, SEXAPLOZZA, Columbus Pride, eXXXotica Tours, House of Bacchus, and Columbus Psych Fest. She is a current columnist for Sexpert.com and *ASN Lifestyle Magazine,* publishing a monthly column mostly regarding mastering your orgasm. Debra has also performed in the global movement entitled "The Vagina Monologues" for three years.

She is the author of over 14 courses, available at shademediallc. com. Five courses are specific to intimacy fulfillment and the other nine are for anyone who wants to become a Sexpert. Taking the courses in the privacy of your home and on your time is a perk, and one of the many quality standards she holds for her course work.

You can find more information about Debra Shade on FB, TW and Insta @shadeyontop.